101

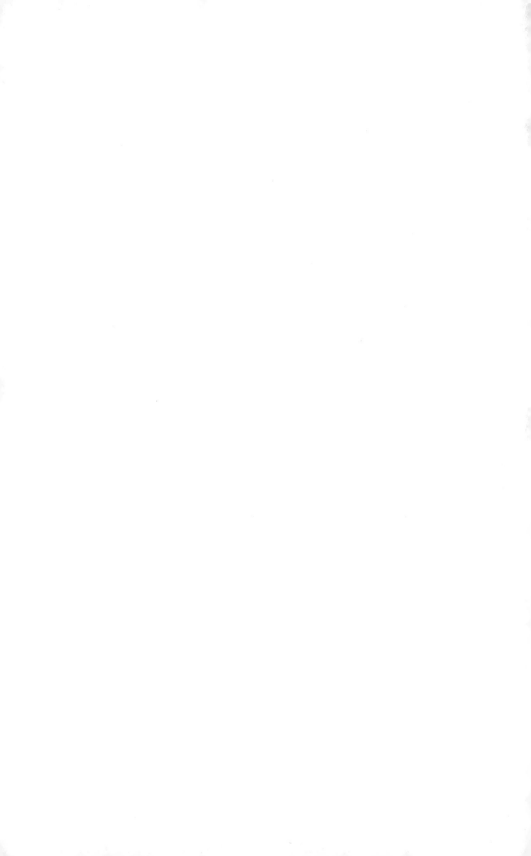

WHY
WE
HURT

OTHER BOOKS BY
FRANK T. VERTOSICK JR., M.D.

When the Air Hits Your Brain

WHY
WE
HURT

The Natural History of Pain

Frank T. Vertosick Jr., M.D.

HARCOURT, INC.

New York   San Diego   London

Library of Congress Cataloging-in-Publication Data

Vertosick, Frank T.
Why we hurt: the natural history of pain / Frank T. Vertosick Jr.
p. cm.
Includes index.
ISBN 0-15-100377-7
1. Pain—Popular works. 2. Pain—History. I. Title.

RB127.V47 2000
616'.0472—dc21 99-045848

Designed by Ivan Holmes
Text set in Janson
Printed in the United States of America

First edition
E D C B A

To Kathy, Emily, and Elizabeth

"friends forever"

Pain as God's Megaphone is
a terrible instrument.

—C. S. Lewis, *The Problem of Pain*

CONTENTS

WHY
WE
HURT

INTRODUCTION
The Megaphone of God

To life, which is the place of pain...

—Bhagavad Gita, chapter VIII

Why do we experience pain?

In the simplest sense, pain protects us from bodily harm. Dangerous things are hurtful things, and pain punishes us if we take excessive risks or push our bodies beyond their physical limits. Fire destroys, fire kills...and so pain teaches us to avoid fire. Without the lessons of pain, our bodies would soon be ravaged by commonplace traumas. Witness the cruel limb deformities seen in numbing diseases such as leprosy and syphilis, and in children with the congenital absence of pain perception.

But this mechanistic definition belies the more mysterious nature of human pain, a nature rooted in something deeper than Darwinian survivalism. From what dangers do migraine headaches and menstrual cramps shield us? Why do harmless colds cause us such misery? Why does childbirth, a natural and essential process, hurt so badly?

Ancient religious teachings equate pain with life itself. The Hindu scripture quoted above, from the Bhagavad Gita, calls life "the place of pain." The Word of Buddha's first sacred truth asserts that life and pain are inseparable: "Birth is suffering; Decay is suffering; Death is suffering;...in short: the Five Groups of Existence are suffering." These are depressing philosophies to be sure, but hardly surprising coming from people living prior to the advent of narcotics, anesthesia, and high-speed dental drills. Nevertheless, the Bhagavad Gita and the Word of Buddha overstate the problem—life and pain are far from synonymous. In fact, most living species experience no pain at all, or at least nothing that we would call pain in the human sense.

Pain is a teacher, the headmaster of nature's survival school, and like any teacher it requires pupils with an ability to learn. Pain's punishments serve no purpose in creatures incapable of recalling bad experiences and using them to modify future behavior. Plants don't feel pain because they have no behaviors to modify; primitive animals such as sponges, worms, and insects don't feel pain because their behaviors are, for the most part, genetically determined. An ant runs from the heat of a flame, but this is instinctive reflex and not learned aversion. A toy robot can be programmed to change direction when it strikes a wall, but this doesn't mean a robot feels pain.

Simple animals with limited behavioral repertoires and life spans numbering in weeks or months enter the world already equipped with the knowledge they need to survive; pain's negative reinforcement would be wasted on them. Pain only matters to organisms with an advanced talent for learning, remembering, and adapting. Buddha's dogma must therefore be reformulated: Pain isn't synonymous with life; it's synonymous with *intelligence*. Cognition of pain, like cognition in general, requires sophisticated neurological hardware.

In plants and lower animals, the preservation of a species requires little in the way of cognitive skills. How smart does a jellyfish need to be? Survival of these species can be assured through the use of heavy armor, redundant anatomy, large-scale reproduction, and other uncomplicated tricks. Since a tree can't withdraw its leaves from a hungry deer, it makes more leaves than it needs. The deer eats its fill and the tree survives. No need for pain here. Likewise, insects, earthworms, and other invertebrates often have spare body parts—extra eyes, wings, and legs—that enable the animals to function even after massive trauma. No need for pain here, either. And lower animals can churn out hundreds, even thousands, of progeny at a time, making any one organism expendable. For plants and primitive animal forms, redundancy and fecundity compensate for insensate stupidity. Because they are buffered against the detrimental effects of trauma, these species have no need for complicated brains or the cognition of pain.

But with the advent of higher intelligence, an entirely new paradigm of survival emerged, one predicated upon the survival of individuals, not on mass production. As organisms acquired the ability to recall their pasts and use this as a template for their futures, they became more skilled at protecting themselves from injury. They could now learn what feels good and what doesn't and tailor their behavior accordingly. This enabled them to shed redundant anatomy, becoming more efficient in the process. Why eat to support two hundred legs when only four will do?

The dynamics of reproduction changed as well. Higher species now could be propagated by a few thousand organisms instead of a few quadrillion. Individuals became less dispensable, their defenses more sophisticated, and their awareness of environmental hazards more acute. While the invertebrate body is like a Japanese Zero plane of World War II vintage—cheap and comparatively defenseless yet able to overwhelm an opponent with sheer numbers—the mammalian body is like the modern F-16 fighter jet. Expensive and inexpendable, the F-16 comes equipped with a dazzling array of warning systems designed to keep each and every plane in the air. In the military vernacular, the F-16 has a high "survivability." As the need for individual survivability in the animal world escalated, so did the need for more sophisticated warning systems, including a more profound appreciation of pain.

A centipede can lose ten legs and walk away, oblivious to its own dismemberment; a grasshopper can continue to eat its prey even as another predator devours its abdomen. But a single broken limb can end a mammal's life in the wild, and each individual could be precious to its species' survival. Possessing few spare animals and even fewer spare body parts, mammals live in terror of the slightest wound. Evolution allowed them to become efficient—and subsequently much more vulnerable—by increasing their fear of bodily injury. Fewer legs and offspring will suffice only if they are exceedingly well cared for.

Homo sapiens, needless to say, tops the list of vulnerable mammals. In one of his more memorable *Far Side* cartoons, Gary Larson depicts two alligators lounging on a riverbank strewn with shredded clothing. One alligator contentedly picks his teeth and muses, "What type of animals were those? No fur, no tough hide, no sharp claws, no big fangs, nothing! Just all soft and pink!" Larson makes a good point; physically, we are wimps. We can't fly, are comparatively weak, possess no talons or other biological weaponry, wear no natural armor, and have little foot speed. Our hearing is poor and our sense of smell is even worse. Our upright posture frees our hands for useful things but also makes us easily seen and prone to falling down. In their peak reproductive period, women can produce just a single infant each year, and a decade or longer will pass before that infant achieves any semblance of independence. We are fragile...and yet the planet groans under the weight of our numbers.

We thrive because our beefy cerebrums allow us to build devices that make us stronger, fleeter, and fiercer than our natural bodies permit. We represent the end product of an evolutionary trend favoring neurological awareness over brute reproductive force. But while this process made us paragons of braininess, it has also made us the Roderick Usher of the animal world.

Usher, protagonist of Edgar Allan Poe's short story "The Fall of the House of Usher," suffers from a degenerative disease that makes his senses hyperacute. Even the finest silk clothing grates on his skin like coarse sandpaper. While we can compensate for our physical frailness with technology, we remain frail. Like Usher, our vulnerability allows little tolerance for the discomforts endured by other creatures. If we don't eat for a day, we become ravenous. We feel comfortable only in a narrow temperature range; we layer our bodies with clothing, encase our feet in protective shoes, and spend much of the day sheltered from the elements. We cook and season our food, deodorize our air, and shield our heads and eyes from the sun. And these aren't modern practices. Humankind has been building homes, donning clothes, roasting meat, and otherwise manipulating the environment to suit itself since the dawn of history. We control our environment not just because we can, but because we *must* out of biological necessity. As the most cognizant of creatures, we are also the most sensitive. Moreover, certain of our physical adaptations—large heads, complex thumbs, upright spines—make us prone to sufferings unique among mammals.

━━✦━━

Our sensitivity goes far beyond the sensation of bodily injury and discomforts, however. In addition to the physical world inhabited by all living creatures, we alone dwell in a parallel world, an abstract realm of thoughts and emotions. It is a "psychic world" posing its own dangers and inflicting its own wounds. Psychic pain can be as great (if not greater) than pain caused by corporeal trauma. Our mind-body dualism bestows upon us the dubious honor of knowing pain in two domains of existence, the physical and the mental. The intersection of these domains, the melding of biological pain with psychic pain, results in that singularly human amalgam known as suffering.

When a dog breaks a leg he feels physical pain, but when a man breaks a leg he will experience both physical *and* psychic pain. The dog knows only that something is wrong; the man, on the other hand, knows much more. He knows that he may be laid up for weeks; that he might need an operation to repair the damaged bone; that he may never enjoy his favorite sport again; that he may lose his job if he's away from work too long. The terrible pain of a broken leg soon merges with the psychic agonies of anger, frustration, worry, and despair. The dog is in pain; the man suffers.

Human beings not only feel pain; they also foresee its consequences, both real and imaginary, a prescience that enhances misery many times over. An elderly woman suffers from a backache not just because it hurts, but because she's afraid it might signify an occult cancer. An executive workaholic frets about his chest pain—maybe it's just heartburn, but he can't be sure. His worrying soon causes him more torment than his chest. The star running back writhes on the field after a knee injury: is it just a bad sprain, or has the anterior cruciate ligament—and his multimillion-dollar future—sustained irreversible damage? Even if our deepest fears prove unfounded, our worrying still worsens the acute and chronic pains of injury and disease.

And we usually fear the worst. As an emergency room doctor, I treated a man brought in by ambulance after he allegedly amputated his thumb with a supermarket meat slicer. The victim, pale and sweating, retched uncontrollably at the very thought of his injury. After removing the large towel that he had blindly wrapped around his hand, I found that he had only sliced a callus from the thumb. The digit wasn't even bleeding. The patient immediately perked up and left, relieved but embarrassed. The immense horsepower of the human brain allows us to do much more than simply experience pain. We embellish it, magnify it, wallow in it, allow it to rule our lives. My humiliated patient had been reduced to a trembling, vomiting wreck by an injury that existed only in his imagination.

In addition to imaginary pains, our brain also allows us to agonize over other hurts we aren't actually feeling at the moment: future pain, past pain, the pain of loved ones. Just knowing I have a root canal tomorrow can harm my quality of life today. And I remember my wife's tears as she watched our screaming infant daughter being stuck with a doctor's needle for the first time. We even cringe at the sight of pain in strangers and can be deeply affected by feigned agony on movie screens. Because we can think and show empathy, the scope of our pain extends far beyond the here and now of our own bodies. It becomes hard to escape pain, even for a day. Everyone has pain in the future to anticipate and pain in family and friends to worry over. Even during the harmless act of flipping through television channels late at night, I have stumbled across a documentary of a child tormented with cancer pain or a movie scene depicting gruesome torture and have been disturbed by the video image for days. Such is the nature of human suffering. No wonder Buddha felt suffering to be synonymous with existence.

Pain is to suffering what sex is to romance. Products of nerve cells and hormones, pain and sex are simply the physiological substrates for deeper metaphysical phenomena. Suffering, like love, requires a human dimension in addition to the raw biology—a dimension of intellect, imagination, emotions, cultural influences, and spiritual beliefs. Because of its human dimension, the perception of pain varies according to each person's culture, religion, and personal makeup. The modern attitude toward pain differs considerably from that of ancient Spartans. A Navy Seal's idea of pain differs from my own. Pain perception also depends upon the state of mind. An arm injury incurred while drunk driving hurts more than the same injury sustained during a gold medal performance in the Olympic giant slalom. Standing on the winner's platform, listening to the national anthem can ease pain; the same can't be said of sitting in a holding cell in some county jail, watching your reputation go down the drain.

⇥

Pain evolved in concert with animal intelligence while suffering needed the next step in neurological development: the advent of consciousness. Buddha's first truth can be further refined: Suffering is synonymous with awareness. Of course, Buddhism is not alone in its preoccupation with suffering. Suffering plays a central role in all religions, illustrating our profound obsession with pain and its consequences, both here and in the "hereafter."

In his book *The Problem of Pain,* theologian C. S. Lewis explores the inseparability of religion and pain by analyzing what he believes to be the ultimate paradox in Judeo-Christianity: Why would a benevolent and all-powerful Maker create a world so saturated with suffering when He could have made it in any way He desired? Lewis argues that God could never command our attention if we lived in an anesthetic world. Without pain, he reasons, people would be so preoccupied with having a good time that they would not heed their Maker nor have any reason to give praise to Him. Pain becomes, in the words of Lewis, the Divine Megaphone through which God speaks to us, calling us to His worship. As anyone who has ever passed a kidney stone well knows, pain does have a way of commanding our attention. Unfortunately, the Megaphone theory makes God akin to a firefighter who commits arson just to play hero by later extinguishing the flames, or like a nurse who poisons patients to feel the joy of resuscitating them afterward. If Lewis is correct, God has the power to create a pain-free existence but will not do so out of fear of being rendered unneeded, ignored, and irrelevant.

The portrayal of pain in religious writings is more subtle than Lewis acknowledges. Pain's role in religion reflects its role in life: Pain is biological, but suffering necessarily arises from cognitive awareness. Only after Adam and Eve eat from the Tree of Knowledge are their "eyes opened" to true suffering. Later, in the New Testament, even Jesus shows a vulnerability to the mental dimension of pain. Although he would die a terrible death on the cross, Christ's greatest suffering took place in the Garden of Gethsemane, where an intense dread of impending torture caused him to sweat blood. An animal can be tortured to death, but only a human being suffers in anticipation of pain. The Bible, like other religious teachings, contains numerous allegories illustrating the mental dimension of pain. To answer Lewis's question, suffering is neither megaphone nor rod of punishment. It is an inevitable consequence of being aware. To be conscious is to suffer, and, in the Christian paradigm, even the Son of God cannot escape this axiom.

The idea that suffering exists above and beyond physical pain also underlies the concept of hell. Hell, or something like it, is an integral part of many religions, including Greek and Roman mythologies, Hinduism, and Christianity. Hell doesn't employ physical pain, since in hell the soul must suffer sans body. Early religions had trouble imagining pure metaphysical suffering and portrayed hell as a place of bodily torture. Ancient Hindus, for example, believed that souls retained an earthly substance that could be tortured according to the sin committed—gluttons to be boiled in oil, offenders of the higher castes to be torn asunder by swines, and so forth.

The modern Christian hell, the one I was taught in Catholic school, represents psychic suffering distilled to its most crystalline form, a form that needs no skin to burn, limbs to crush, or bowels to tear away. Hell symbolizes the feeling of loss, the feeling of never seeing God or knowing bliss. Hell is not the pain of a broken neck, but the mourning and despair felt by the quadriplegic long after the neck heals. Dante understood this hell. The portal to his Inferno carries the admonition: "Abandon all hope, ye who enter here!" It is this distilled suffering, this hell of earth, that I see in my office every day. Pain that patients suffer not just from their peculiar afflictions, but also from abandonment of their hope for future recovery.

There is a very good reason for understanding the dual nature of pain. The therapy of chronic pain syndromes may require treatment aimed independently at both the mental and physical aspects of suffering. The clinician must acknowledge that these are separable phenomena in many patients and act accordingly. In many cases, suffering can be relieved even though the physical pain that provokes it remains incurable. It is essential for both patient and physician to understand that the treatment of chronic pain extends beyond the limits of biological medicine.

This book contains portraits of human pain and suffering; portraits I have created that are based on real-life experience. It is both a treatise on clinical pain syndromes and an exploration of how those syndromes alter the lives of their victims. It is an anthology of pain patients, the view of clinical hell as seen through the eyes of the damned—but with a crucial difference from real hell: many of the people I depict here found a way out.

Philosopher Bertrand Russell condemns religions that believe in hell, labeling them "ferocious" for even thinking there could be torment without end. He was right; the idea of eternal pain must certainly be the most ferocious thing ever conceived by the human mind, and that's exactly what many chronic pain patients fear most: pain without end. Clinical suffering depends less upon the magnitude of the hurting and more upon the uncertainty over how long the hurting will last. Stepping on a nail or bruising one's shin can cause great physical discomfort, but we know these are fleeting miseries of no permanent consequence. The elderly man with an arthritic spine, on the other hand, fears that he may never feel good again in his lifetime. Although his backache may be minor compared to the pain of an acutely traumatized shinbone, its perpetuity may drive him to the brink of suicide.

In this book I will examine the nature of biological pain in its myriad manifestations: not the transient hurts of bruised shins, paper cuts, or sprained ankles, but the deeper pains caused by childbirth, cancer, and arthritis. I will explore maladies that appear to exist only to push the envelope of our endurance—disorders like postherpetic neuralgia, tic douloureux, diabetic neuropathy, rheumatoid arthritis, and phantom pain. These syndromes are like plants that take their roots in physical pain but grow and flower in the psyches of the afflicted until they choke the joy of life right out of them.

The real mandate of medical care is not the saving of lives, but the dispensing of comfort. We cannot expect to live forever, not yet anyway. However, we *can* hope to live lives free of suffering. That goal may be within our grasp. Fortunately, intelligence is a double-edged sword—while it enables us to perceive suffering, intelligence also gives us the tools to understand and treat the biological processes that give rise to that suffering.

To win any war, one must know the enemy, and great strides have been made in this regard. Afflictions like tic douloureux, phantom pain, and migraine are no longer the enigmas they once were. Likewise, medical science is making rapid progress in the pharmacology of pain relief; more precise methods of drug delivery—from intranasal sprays for the treatment of headaches to the computerized installation of morphine directly into the nervous system for the palliation of cancer pain—are becoming commonplace in clinical practice. The search for newer pain relievers continues. The next candidate drug coming from, of all places, the skin of a frog.

Technical innovations in the field of neurosurgery have revolutionized the surgical treatment of pain. Pain centers in the brain and spinal cord can be destroyed with precision lasers or using microprocessor-guided radiotherapy. Complex electrical stimulators can be inserted directly into the nervous system to mask pain pathways, and gene therapy lies just over the horizon.

Not all pain research has been in the "hard sciences." Interest in the mind-body aspect of suffering has exploded, and therapies aimed at the interface between physical pain and psychic suffering are being subjected to greater scrutiny. Alternative medical approaches to pain—including relaxation therapy, therapeutic touch, massage therapy, and acupuncture—have become big business. In recognition of the roles played by depression and anxiety in chronic pain, conventional psychiatric therapy is also being tried. Some of these approaches look promising; others may prove little more than lucrative pseudoscience.

Although many of the diseases I portray will seem hellish at first, most of the victims did not suffer forever. This book contains some success stories, or at least qualified success stories. Of course, not all chronic pain patients can expect success; no medical discipline, conventional or alternative, will master suffering in all patients at all times. But the odds of success are improving.

Pain is not a punishment from God but a natural process. Sometimes, as in childbirth, pain is unavoidable and must be managed directly. Other times it occurs when our natural pain reflexes become diseased; in these cases, the underlying illnesses can often be ameliorated or cured through timely intervention.

The case histories that I've created here illustrate how even people trapped in a living Inferno can emerge to lead normal lives again.

This book is about the biological nature of pain and our attempts to expunge it from our lives. Nearly all of us will fall victim to some form of chronic pain; by understanding the beast, we will be better equipped to grapple with it.

When treating pain, knowledge is still the best weapon.

1 HEAD PAINS AND CANDY CANES

I know that pain is to be fought and thrown aside, not to be accepted as part of one's soul and as a permanent scar across one's existence.

—John Galt, in Ayn Rand's *Atlas Shrugged*

I'd like to begin the story of pain on a personal note. I was about twelve or thirteen years old when my headaches began—and I use the word *headache* with some reluctance. Although it's the commonly accepted word, *headache* is entirely too meek a term for my condition. *Webster's Dictionary* defines an ache as a "dull, persistent pain" and that's not what I was feeling in my head. What I felt was persistent all right, but not dull—*explosive* and *incapacitating* would be better adjectives.

I never had headaches during school hours, only at home and usually on the weekends. They would last for hours at a time, forcing me to lie in a darkened room with a trash can at my side for the inevitable vomiting while my friends enjoyed Little League baseball or cruised our suburban roadways on their bikes. Fortunately, the headaches rarely happened more than once or twice a month and I never considered myself ill.

Of course, my parents thought otherwise. They hauled me to a pediatrician, an ENT specialist, and an ophthalmologist, in search of a diagnosis. Like all concerned parents, they feared the worst—a brain tumor—but these doctors gave us no answers, good or bad. I did need glasses, as it turned out, but correcting my vision didn't change things. I was diagnosed with hay fever, too, but the prescribed antihistamines just made me dopey and did nothing to reduce the frequency or severity of the headaches. Had the year been 1998, instead of 1968, doctors would have scanned my brain immediately. Alas, CT or MRI scanners didn't exist thirty years ago, not even on paper. In those Dark Ages of medicine, physicians would never think to subject an otherwise healthy young boy to the pain and terror of cerebral angiography and pneumoencephalography—the only brain images obtainable in my childhood—simply because he had an occasional bad headache. I'm still alive thirty years later, and so the decision not to torture me looking for a nonexistent brain tumor was a wise one (and one for which I remain eternally grateful).

A family doctor offered me a rather lame diagnosis: chronic headaches. His therapeutic advice was equally vague and useless: take aspirin. I had already told him that aspirin never helped, but he shrugged and offered no additional suggestions. Like many chronic pain patients, my therapy quickly became my personal responsibility. I was left to decipher my illness and devise my own coping strategies, which I did.

But it took me almost twenty years.

Three decades and a medical degree later, I now know that I suffer from migraines, a ferocious form of episodic headache that afflicts almost one in five adults to some degree. *Migraine* is a weird corruption of the word *hemicranial,* meaning "half of the head." Migraines typically affect only one side of the head at a time, right or left, while other forms of headache involve both sides equally. Migraines also prefer the front of the head, including the face, in contrast to tension headaches (also called muscular headaches), which localize to the back of the head or upper neck. Headaches caused by brain tumors or hemorrhages radiate to the very top of the head or may even be perceived in the entire head. Moreover, tumor headaches are usually associated with mental aberrations—somnolence, confusion, memory lapses—abnormalities rarely seen in migraine patients. My own pain affected my eyes, forehead, nose, and nasal sinuses—usually on the right side—a distribution fairly typical of migraine.

How to describe the severity of a migraine? A close friend of mine, a nephrologist practicing in Florida, teases me by saying that migraines are just routine headaches that occur in wimps. He is, needless to say, quite wrong. The severity of migraines stems from the magnitude of the pain, not from the oversensitivity of the afflicted. The best way to simulate a migraine is to drink a cold milk shake very quickly. This maneuver will induce the bizarre phenomenon known variously as "ice-cream headache," "brain freeze," or "cold head," a penetrating sensation that grips the frontal sinuses, eyes, and forehead like a vise, often causing a person to wince and pinch the bridge of the nose until the pain eases. Now imagine having that "brain freeze" pain not for the usual ten seconds but for *three hours.* That's a migraine.

When migraines reach a crescendo, sufferers must put forth a Herculean effort to do anything, even routine things like walking, talking, or keeping their eyes open. Thinking becomes virtually impossible. Using one's brain to perform complex tasks during a migraine is like trying to run on a broken leg. It just can't be done, no matter how determined the thinker or runner might be. Migraine victims wish only to slink away and retire to bed, far from everybody and everything. The pain, aided by derangements in the nervous system, also causes severe nausea and reflexive vomiting.

In the 1998 Super Bowl, a star running back had to sit out a portion of the game because of a migraine—imagine the headache that could keep a player out of *that* arena. All due respects to my Florida friend, but professional football players do not generally qualify as wimps. I was watching a recent professional golf tournament, and the golfer who was leading the field almost pulled out during the last round because of his migraine. He struggled through and went on to win, yet he almost traded $700,000 for a chance to go and lie down. These examples put some perspective on how bad the pain can be.

The great Pittsburgh hockey player Mario Lemieux endured recurring bouts of severe back spasms during his career, the result of a degenerating disc and a postoperative spine infection. During one particularly bad episode—when he couldn't bend over to tie his shoes let alone play a contact sport—a young television reporter asked him why he couldn't simply "play through" his pain. I'll never forget the incredulous look on the All-Star center's normally stoic face as he replied indignantly: "I just can't." I knew exactly what Lemieux was thinking. Unless you've endured the pain, you simply cannot understand. Migraine sufferers (more elegantly known as migraineurs) know Lemieux's indignation. There are some pains that even the strongest of us cannot "play through."

Migraines belong to a broader category of pain syndromes known as vascular headaches, which include common migraine, classic migraine, ophthalmoplegic migraine, basilar migraine, and a rare but ruthless disease that affects mostly elderly men known as cluster headache. Vascular headaches are so named because their pain emanates from arteries supplying blood to the scalp, dura (the inner lining of the skull), and brain. A vascular headache consists of two separate phases: an arterial constriction phase and an arterial dilation phase.

During the constriction phase, blood vessels narrow in response to a chemical hormone called serotonin. Serotonin is in the class of compounds known as neurotransmitters; also in this category of substances are dopamine, the neurotransmitter involved in schizophrenia and Parkinson's disease, and epinephrine (more commonly called adrenaline). Serotonin is secreted after the susceptible person is exposed to a headache "trigger" that may be contained in certain foods, especially red wine, cheeses, and bean products. Other headache triggers include caffeine or monosodium glutamate, allergens (pollen, dust mites), hormonal changes, head trauma, psychic stresses, severe exertion, and prolonged sleeplessness.

During the arterial constriction phase, narrowing of the arteries restricts blood flow to the scalp and brain. This phase is painless, although the sluggish blood flow to the brain may cause the migraineur to feel odd sensations known as migrainous auras. Auras can take many forms: feelings of anxiety, dizziness, out-of-body experiences, distorted spatial perception. Simple visual hallucinations are most common. On the very rarest of occasions, reduced blood flow during a migraine can even lead to a stroke.

After the arterial constriction ends, a second phase occurs wherein arteries suddenly dilate and become engorged with blood. This dilation may be the brain's attempt to overcompensate for the reduced blood flow that occurred during the arterial constriction phase, akin to a starving man ordering up an eight-course meal. A migraineur feels headache pain during the dilation phase as sensitive arterial walls stretch to twice their normal size. The arteries derive their nerve supply from the upper branches of the trigeminal nerve, the nerve that supplies sensation to the forehead and eyes. This wiring transmits the pain of arterial stretching predominantly to the eyes and upper face. Migraines are first cousins to another debilitating condition to be discussed later: trigeminal neuralgia, or tic douloureux; migraines and tic are both cephalgias mediated by the trigeminal nerve.

Because migraine pain originates in the arteries, the pain can be worsened by turning the head, which stretches the aching arterial walls further. The pain also fluctuates in frequency and severity with the beating of the heart. A rapid, bounding pulse will make the pain of migraines worse, something I can confirm from personal experience. Anything that increases the robustness and rate of the heart's rhythm will accentuate the pain. That's why I, like other migraineurs, try to keep as quiet and motionless as possible during an attack. Years ago, when forced to run to a toilet because of acute nausea, my heart rate jumped so high that I thought the arterial pounding would blow off the top of my head. I've tried not to repeat that mistake.

The dilation phase persists for several hours, although a few misfortunates have headaches lasting several days. After the acute pain subsides, the victim is often left with a dull but tolerable throbbing in the head and a feeling of complete exhaustion.

Not every migraineur has an aura during the constriction phase; among headache syndromes, however, aura is unique to migraines. Because of the aura, migraines have become something of a romantic affliction almost epidemic in the artistically inclined, like tuberculosis was a century ago. The auras of famous migraineurs have become the stuff of legend. The macabre world of *Alice in Wonderland* sprang from the spatial distortions experienced by Lewis Carroll during his auras. The oil paintings of De Chirico likewise show the influence of his migrainous hallucinations. Nietzsche was nearly driven mad by headaches—although his tertiary syphilis didn't help matters—and who knows what insights the philosopher gained from his auras. Some authors, including neurologist Oliver Sacks, have even suggested that some famous religious "visions" may have been auras as well.

The romantic association between migraines and intellectuals at one time had some basis in science. Migraines were once thought to be more common in the mentally gifted, a belief supported by limited epidemiological evidence. This idea has been refuted by more recent studies showing no relationship between migraines and intelligence.

Times change, and auras are no longer the artistic fad they once were. Altered mental states induced by illicit drugs can do the same job as auras for people looking to draw their inspiration from deranged brain chemistry—although I doubt that *Alice in Wonderland* would have had the same quaint charm had it been conceived on LSD. It's just as well that migraines are no longer romanticized; I never found my headaches particularly inspiring. To a migraineur, headaches aren't the engines of De Chirico oils, Carroll fables, or beatific visions of the Virgin Mary. They are instruments of torment, nothing more or less.

Their supposed artistic impact aside, auras do serve a useful role for the migraineur: they sound a warning, alerting the victim that a headache is on the way. Auras are the distant rumblings of a freight train about to crash into your head. To use an aura as a warning sign, however, the victim has to recognize that it is, in fact, an aura. This sounds silly—can a migraineur really be unaware of an aura? In fact, yes; recognizing auras is not always easy.

The word *aura* is from the Latin word for "gentle breeze," and that's exactly what an aura can be: gentle. Not all auras are as dramatic as those that inspired Alice's sojourn down a rabbit hole; most auras are subtle and easy to ignore, consisting of brief visual disturbances. Since flashing spots, afterimages, and "floaters" can affect anybody's vision from time to time—particularly now that half our waking hours are spent welded to video games and computer monitors—the average migraineur may not recognize the hallucinations as a sign of imminent headache. In my own case, years of headaches came and went before I realized that I was having auras.

My own aura takes the form of a tiny iridescent candy cane twirling slowly in the extreme lower right of my peripheral vision. The candy cane becomes visible only if I stare at an empty wall or blank sheet of paper. I can't look at it directly since it immediately shifts away like a mischievous imp dancing at the limits of my vision. (I have also lost large sections of my vision for an hour or more during an aura; while this sounds frightening, those of us with a long history of classic migraines learn to expect such nuisances from time to time.)

Recognizing my own unique aura was one step toward conquering my headaches; this recognition took me a very long time, largely because I didn't know that such things as auras even existed. During the first decade of my migraines, I knew very little about my illness and did nothing to learn more about it, a stupid approach for anyone with a chronic disease. The fact that my headaches were relatively infrequent by most migraine standards also made it difficult for me to identify patterns in their behavior.

I still recall the day I realized that my body was alerting me to a looming migraine. I was in college. While reclining on my bed after a grueling organic chemistry test, I began staring mindlessly at the white plaster ceiling above (this was during my childless days, when lying motionless on a bed in the middle of the day was actually possible). I remember seeing a little candy cane, bright as a neon beer sign in a tavern window. It was a radiant rod of spinning, twinkling light made of pink and white stripes and rotating on its axis about once a second. What an interesting hallucination, I thought, but what the hell is it? Having survived the '60s and '70s without so much as smoking a cigarette, I wondered if this is the sort of vision that drugs can induce. I watched it for a while, then called a friend and made plans to go eat at a fast-food place. I never made it; the rest of my day was spent sick in bed with a terrible headache.

That event was an epiphany for me. Ignorant as I was of brain matters at that time in my life, I knew that there had to be some connection between the bizarre illusion and the headache. My brain was waving this candy cane at me like a semaphore flag signaling of danger ahead. The possibility that the candy cane was a migrainous omen had crossed my mind even before the headache began; previous experience taught me that my migraines often happened after a stressful event, like my organic chemistry test. I was expecting a headache even before the candy cane appeared.

By the time I finished college, I had an excellent notion of what would bring on a severe headache and the various forms my auras would take. Unfortunately, I still hadn't figured out how to stop the migraines entirely. The aura was still useful, for whenever I saw the candy cane I knew I had to cancel my immediate plans and hide out in my bedroom. I experimented with what methods I had available before finally finding the solution with a simple over-the-counter medication. Seeking professional help never occurred to me, strangely enough—a big mistake for today's migraineur.

Early in the course of my disease, I learned that if I fell asleep just after a headache arrived, I could stop it. Sometimes I needed to sleep for only five or ten minutes to get rid of the pain. It wasn't foolproof—sometimes I often awoke with a headache— but it worked well enough that sleep became my first line of defense. Sometimes sleeping just wasn't possible—for example, if I got an aura while driving (although I did pull off an interstate once to fall asleep sitting up in my car).

Most of the time, unfortunately, I just couldn't sleep because the headache was just too intense. Once the headache began, I was stuck in a catch-22 situation: I couldn't relieve the headache without falling asleep and I couldn't fall asleep as long as the headache was there. Victims of any chronic pain syndrome know that lying down to sleep can be the hardest time of the day. To fall asleep, one needs to free the mind of distractions; but for chronic pain patients, distractions may be the only thing that keeps the pain at bay. As we try to sleep, we end up giving pain our full, undivided attention and the pain usually makes the most of it.

Unaware that there were good drugs for stopping migraines, I tried bizarre and dangerous things to get enough temporary relief to fall asleep. I even tried taking twenty-five aspirin tablets at once (an overdose, but I didn't know that then). Two pills never worked, so why not try half a bottle? I learned firsthand the horrors of cinchonism, a temporary affliction named for the bark of the cinchona tree, the natural source of aspirin. The hallmark of cinchonism is tinnitus, an unbearable high-pitched whine in the ears caused by chemical irritation of the auditory nerves. The tinnitus lasted for hours and I thought I would go mad. The experience made me swear off pills for years, which was also a mistake.

One day I made a very utilitarian—albeit somewhat disgusting—observation: if I vomited, my headache pain abated briefly, sometimes for almost ten blissful minutes. Based on this serendipitous observation, I soon developed a ritual of vomiting followed by hurriedly lying down and trying to fall asleep. If I didn't fall asleep within this eye of the migrainous hurricane, my headache returned, making it impossible to sleep; I would be forced to repeat the process. It would often take five or more such cycles of vomiting and resting before I managed to doze off. More often than not, I wound up asleep next to some toilet, stiff and sore but headache free.

This trick worked well for migraines that made me nauseated, but sometimes I didn't feel nauseated. What then? I quickly developed ways of making myself vomit, with or without nausea. During my college years, when my headaches came as often as once or twice a week, I developed a freakish ability to throw up without any provocation and on a moment's notice. In *Angela's Ashes*, Pulitzer Prize–winning author Frank McCourt describes with awe a man from his destitute Irish neighborhood who could imbibe ale for hours and then heave it back up without so much as putting a finger down his throat. This man was a hero to the local pub crawlers. I think I would have been a god in McCourt's neighborhood.

After I finished medical school, I met a hairdresser who also used self-induced vomiting to treat her migraines. She had to stop the practice after a bad bout of retching detached one of her retinas and blinded her in the right eye. This frightened me, needless to say, but I didn't know what else to do. By then I had relied on vomiting for years; it worked very well and I knew of no other way to abort the pain so quickly. It was still nice to meet a kindred spirit, nice to know that I wasn't the only one driven to using extreme pain control measures.

Although research continues to unravel *how* vascular headaches occur, we still have little insight into *why* they occur. There must be some biological reason for these headaches given their ubiquitous nature. Unlike pain syndromes stemming from the aging process (for example, trigeminal neuralgia and osteoarthritis), migraines usually begin at or before the age of puberty. Moreover, vascular headaches have a strong genetic component. Most migraineurs have an immediate family member who also suffers from the disease.

Common genetic diseases that onset prior to the peak childbearing years usually provide some selective survival advantage from an evolutionary standpoint, otherwise they would not be propagated from generation to generation. And we know vascular headaches are not a recent affliction; the first descriptions of the disease date back five thousand years. The Peruvian trephinations—ancient South American skulls bearing healed surgical openings—may represent early attempts to treat chronic headaches by letting "evil spirits" escape from the brain.

Anatomically, the nerve centers that give rise to headaches are situated deep within the most ancient parts of the brain, the hypothalamus and brain stem, evidence that headaches have been around for a very long time, perhaps since the evolution of the head itself. Thus, we can conclude that migraines represent an ancient phenomenon genetically imprinted into the brain's core wiring for thousands, maybe even millions, of years. But for what purpose?

After all, migraineurs should be at a selective *disadvantage* for survival compared to nonmigraineurs, a fact that runs contrary to the grain of evolution. While evolutionary pressures don't matter for degenerative illnesses that limit the survival of the elderly, they would certainly come to bear on a common debilitating condition affecting the very young. Lying helpless with a devastating headache for many hours couldn't have been a safe behavior for primitive humans. Migraineurs would have been more prone to being devoured by wild beasts. Or spurned by their societies as nonproductive malingerers (which happens even today). Or even executed as hopelessly demon possessed.

As mysterious as evolution can be, however, it isn't stupid. Migraines must serve some beneficial function that compensates for their transient periods of dangerous incapacity, else the genetic predisposition for headaches would have been cleansed from our gene pool long ago. In truth, quite the opposite is occurring: not only are headache syndromes extraordinarily common, some studies suggest that they are increasing in prevalance over time.

Perhaps migraines are *supposed* to incapacitate us, at least temporarily. There is ample precedent for using transient incapacity as a survival strategy. The very act of sleeping may be one example. Some theorists believe that sleep does nothing but keep us out of trouble for a few hours. A less controversial example can be found in our response to infectious diseases like the flu.

The influenza virus only wants to borrow our bodies for a week or two so that it can use our cells' enzymatic factories to produce progeny. There is no reason why an influenza infestation should make us feel miserable, but it does. During a viral infection, our immune system releases hormones that give us fever, make us ache, cause us to shiver uncontrollably, and, in general, force us to crawl into some hole until it all goes away. The virus doesn't make us sick; our immune systems make us *feel* sick in response to acute infection. Like migraines, the pain and malaise of viral infections are self-induced miseries.

There is a Darwinian rationale for our masochistic response to pathogens like the flu: containing the spread of infection. Although a flu virus doesn't set out to kill us, occasionally that does happen. From a survival advantage, it's best not to get the flu. Since primitive humans knew nothing about germ theory and had no intellectual motivation to avoid each other during viral outbreaks, the body had to come up with a way of containing the contagion and it did so by making viral illnesses physically incapacitating. Flu sufferers become so tired, sore, and wretched that they feel compelled to go off by themselves until the contagious period passes.

Even in the modern era, this ancient survival strategy works well. Sick children are less likely to go to school and infect other children. Sick adults stay out of the workplace and feel less inclined to socialize. If the flu didn't make us feel ill, there would be no behavioral barriers to this viral transmission.

But migraines aren't contagious, so what useful purpose would their pain-induced incapacity serve? Although the tendency to have migraines is inherited, the headaches themselves are triggered by some stimulus—foods, toxins, stress, sleeplessness, hormonal surges. Perhaps migraines represent an adaptive response to one of these triggering stimuli. The primordial role of pain is that of a teacher, an instructor in the ways of survival. If that's so, what lesson are migraines trying to teach us?

One possibility: Migraines may be nature's way of telling us to avoid certain foods, toxins, or allergens in the environment. Although it is an attractive theory, I find it untenable. Even with modern clinical monitoring, identifying what foods or allergens trigger a given migraineur's headaches can take months of investigation, and in many cases an environmental trigger is never found. The association of migraines with external triggers like food or allergens is far too subtle for the headaches to serve as a natural form of aversion training. Besides, our bodies can employ more immediate and direct methods of informing us when we have eaten something bad or have been exposed to some allergen—for example, vomiting, diarrhea, itching, wheezing.

The evolution of migraines may have more to do with intrinsic triggers—stress and hormonal changes—than with environmental triggers. The link between migraines and sex hormones may be of particular importance. Of all known migraine triggers, female sex hormones—estrogen and progesterone—are the most potent. Older preparations of oral contraceptives that used high doses of these hormones were notorious for exacerbating migraines in known migraineurs, and even inducing migraine syndromes in women who never had headaches before starting the drugs.

In adolescence, migraines affect boys and girls equally. However, the incidence of migraines increases more rapidly in women. Female migraineurs eventually outnumber males three to one. Moreover, the frequency and severity of headaches in women is intimately related to their menstrual cycles, pregnancy status, and onset of menopause.

Headaches often cycle with menstruation ("menstrual migraine"); they also increase in frequency during the first trimester of pregnancy. And while migraine frequency in men diminishes with age, in women headaches may worsen after the onset of menopause. These observations suggest a pivotal role for female sex hormones in the pathogenesis of vascular headaches. It's tempting to speculate that migraines might have something to do with sexual behavior, particularly with the timing of sexual intercourse relative to the ovulatory cycle. Although "Not tonight, dear, I have a headache" has become a cliché, headaches may serve as a crude regulator of intercourse frequency. Female migraines occur most commonly during periods of peak infertility—just before, during, and after menstruation; during pregnancy, especially in the first trimester when conception is not externally apparent; and after menopause.

Humans are relatively unique among primates in that our ovulation occurs silently. In other words, we don't come into "heat." During ovulation in baboons, females undergo anatomic changes and develop a ravenous appetite for indiscriminant sex, copulating with any available male. When not ovulating, she has no interest in intercourse whatsoever and males have no interest in her. Humans, being ignorant of the moment of ovulation, must engage in a lower frequency of intercourse scattered randomly throughout the ovulatory cycle. As we will see later, this unique reproductive physiology comes into play in other painful events, including childbirth, menstruation, and menopause.

As Jared Diamond and other physiologists have argued, the fact that we don't come into heat doesn't mean that the timing of human sexual intercourse is left entirely to chance, devoid of all biological regulation. In baboons, the timing of intercourse is determined by positive reinforcement—a sudden, intense desire to copulate. In humans, the timing seems most influenced by negative reinforcement—the intense desire *not* to copulate. The severe nausea experienced in early pregnancy, the pains caused by menstruation and menopause, the very fact that women menstruate at all (as opposed to reabsorbing their uterine lining entirely) may all be natural means of inhibiting intercourse during periods of peak infertility. In this context, migraines may be just another method of engineering sexual behavior to maximize fecundity.

We also cannot easily discount the influence of psychic stress in vascular headache syndromes. In my case, stress was the only reliable trigger that I could identify. Interestingly, migraines typically occur after stressful events, not before or during such events. My migraines never happened at school or during major tests but many hours later. I also never worried about getting a migraine while performing surgery—that's never happened in twenty years—although I have gotten an occasional attack after long and challenging surgeries. Clearly, migraines could not serve as a survival mechanism if they incapacitated us when we absolutely *had* to do something. There have been one or two instances when I was called upon to do emergency surgery just as I felt a migraine brewing. I simply willed the headache away.

Migraines may be an adaptive mechanism forcing us to rest after a harrowing experience. Ancient humans might have gotten so pumped up after killing their first mastodon that they would run off and do something stupid. A bad headache would inhibit that. Migraines are like a stern but benevolent parent telling us we've been through enough and should attempt to do no more for a while.

The association of migraines with stressful situations is more obvious to the average migraineur than any associations with external factors such as foods. Thus, while migraines would be a poor form of aversive training for foods, they might be a good way of teaching us to avoid conflicts and stresses that might harm us in other ways.

One final possibility: The headaches themselves may give us no survival advantage, but the genetic predisposition to headaches just might. I know this sounds confusing, but there are numerous examples of a genetic predisposition to disease offering a survival advantage even though the disease itself is harmful or deadly. Consider sickle cell anemia.

Sickle cell anemia is a blood disease common in African Americans. In sickle cell disease, the normally round red blood cells become deformed into nonfunctioning sickle-shaped cells, hence the name. People who get a single copy of the sickle cell gene from one parent have what is known as sickle cell trait and exhibit a mild asymptomatic deformity of their blood cells. People who carry two copies, one from each parent, get full-blown anemia and often die in childhood or early adolescence.

Sickle cell trait is very common in black Americans and even more so in native African populations, yet the overt anemia it causes is lethal. We have now learned that people with sickle cell trait are immune to malaria, the most common infectious killer in Africa. Thus, a mild predisposition to sickle cell anemia offers a survival advantage—malarial resistance—that saves more lives than will be lost to the full-blown disease. Even though sickle anemia is a killer, sickle cell trait has allowed the continued human presence in a malaria-infested continent. A little bit of the sickle cell gene is good—too much is very, very bad.

Similarly, full-blown cystic fibrosis is lethal, yet the mild genetic predisposition to Cf may protect against typhoid and cholera. Full-blown Tay-Sachs disease, a neurological disorder endemic in Jewish populations, is also lethal, but a mild genetic predisposition to Tay-Sachs may protect against tuberculosis. Perhaps people like me—with full-blown migraines—may have two copies of some beneficial gene, a gene that confers a survival advantage on a headache-free population possessing only one copy.

➤

For whatever reason, whether simple bad luck or crafty evolutionary genetics, migraines remain a thorny problem for modern humankind. Today's migraineurs shouldn't follow my bad example; they should instead seek the advice of a qualified neurologist early on. Better yet, a number of major cities now have dedicated "headache centers" that offer a variety of diagnostic, therapeutic, and lifestyle management options.

As a first step in treating migraines, a certain diagnosis of benign vascular headache should be made and other causes of headache should be ruled out. Although everyone fears a brain tumor, life-threatening conditions such as meningitis, tumors, or hemorrhages account for less than 1 percent of all chronic head pains. More common maladies masquerading as migraines include glaucoma, trigeminal neuralgia, temporal arteritis, dysfunction of the temporomandibular (jaw) joint, and sinus disease. The body can be wired in strange ways and any number of diseases can cause severe headaches. I have cared for people with cardiac disease, ruptured neck discs, chronic carbon monoxide poisoning, and carpal tunnel disease who were mistakenly believed to have migraines.

Once the diagnosis of migraine has been established, simple lifestyle modifications should be tried first. Common food triggers like caffeine, red wine, chocolate, beans, and cheese should be reduced or eliminated one at a time. It may also help to stop smoking since the carbon monoxide in cigarette smoke can worsen headaches. It also helps to limit stress, but that's easier said than done.

Oral contraceptives, if being used at the time headaches first occur, should be stopped temporarily. Oddly enough, in some women contraceptives actually relieve the headache, although using estrogen products to treat migraines remains somewhat controversial. Some neurologists believe that the risk of migraine-related stroke is increased by concurrent use of sex hormones.

If these modifications fail and the headaches occur fre- quently, most neurologists will prescribe a headache-suppressing drug like propranolol, amitriptyline, or valproate. These prophy- lactic drugs must be taken daily for years and, although generally safe, should not be given to migraineurs who have headaches only rarely.

Prophylactic drugs aren't analgesics; they reduce the fre- quency of headaches but have no benefit once a headache begins. Although a variety of powerful prescription drugs have become available for aborting a headache in progress, many migraines will still respond to inexpensive over-the-counter analgesics like aspirin, acetaminophen, or ibuprofen when taken in sufficient doses. I was thirty-five years old and a migraineur for over twenty years when I discovered that a gram of acetaminophen taken im- mediately after an aura would block the ensuing headache virtu- ally every time. I now keep a bottle of the children's chewable variety everywhere—in my office, my car, the operating room— and I haven't had a migraine, or a vomiting episode, in over five years.

Why didn't I try this common drug years earlier? Because I fell victim to two myths endemic among migraineurs: (1) strong headaches require strong (prescription) medications; and (2) if one over-the-counter medication fails (as aspirin did for me), all such medications will fail. Neither conclusion is valid.

Different people respond to any medication differently and nonprescription drugs are no exception. Acetaminophen may work beautifully for one person but not at all for another. Each person must try a variety of over-the-counter preparations at their maximum safe doses and try them several times before deciding that prescription drugs are necessary.

Sometimes the strongest medications aren't the best medications. Curiously, powerful narcotics, particularly morphine and codeine, frequently fail to help migraines and occasionally worsen them. Furthermore, narcotics tend to be short-lived, too short-lived to last for an entire headache, and they pose too great an addictive risk for people suffering from a decades-long illness.

The most effective migraine-abortive prescription medications include drugs that constrict throbbing blood vessels (for example, ergotamine) and drugs like sumatriptan that interfere with serotonin, the chemical thought to be responsible for the headaches in the first place. These drugs pack a wallop and must be taken with caution, especially in patients with other forms of vascular disease. Excessive use of ergotamine, for example, may cause vascular constriction in the extremities and can lead to gangrene of the toes and fingers, a most unpleasant side effect.

A variety of other treatment approaches have been tried over the years, including dripping local anesthetics into the nose or eyes, acupuncture, chiropractic manipulation of the head and neck (which recent evidence suggests is worthless), biofeedback, aromatherapy, massage, psychotherapy, and some therapies too bizarre to mention here. Suffice it to say that most migraineurs will eventually develop some coping strategy, as I did, but only after a long period of trial and error and a lot of effort (and grief) on the part of the migraineur. Final control of the headaches may require an assault on a number of fronts simultaneously, and most severe migraineurs employ an eclectic mix of dietary changes, stress management, prophylactic drugs, abortive drugs, and a few personalized behaviors (like my circus geek–like gastronomical control) to stay pain free.

One last personal note: John Galt's quote at the beginning of this chapter carries an important lesson—pain should not be a permanent scar on our souls. Rand's golden-haired superman lived a life immune to "fear, guilt or pain," but the same can't be said for the rest of us. We all face fear, guilt, and pain in abundance. We can't eliminate them, but we can do our best not to let these things rule our lives.

I was determined not to let my headaches interfere with my career. In fact, no one outside of my family knew that I had migraines, until medical school. While on a skiing trip with some fellow students, I fell on an icy slope during the first run of the day, hitting my head on the hard ground. I subsequently developed such a severe headache that I was forced to spend the rest of the long day lying on the wet, freezing floor of the ski lodge's men's room. I was forced to confess my headache tendency to my friends, who couldn't help but notice my prolonged absence and pale appearance.

One student got a puzzled look on her face and asked me if I wasn't afraid of entering a long surgical residency with a history of debilitating migraines. This took me by surprise—I hadn't even thought of that before. What if I got a migraine while on call or in the OR? After a brief wave of panic, I simply replied no. I would manage somehow.

And so I have.

2 SLAYING THE PHANTOM

*I felt my head and breast to satisfy myself whether
it was I myself who was there, or some empty,
elusive phantom...*

—Miguel de Cervantes,
Don Quixote

During the last century and the first half of this century, many physicians thought that chronic pain could be cured by cutting nerves. If the face hurt, surgeons cut the nerves to the face; if the arm hurt, they severed the nerves to the arm; and so on. This rendered the skin numb, of course, and sometimes even caused paralysis, but patients and doctors alike believed that numbness and weakness would be preferable to a lifetime of pain. They were wrong. Although patients might be better temporarily, a worse fate awaited them months and years later. To understand why cutting nerves doesn't relieve pain and may, in fact, worsen it, consider the case of Rich McKnight.

Dr. Rich McKnight worked as an anesthesiologist at one of our local community hospitals. In his midthirties and recently divorced, Rich lived the life of the single male blessed with a large income and good looks. He lifted weights, frequented nightclubs, and rode a jet black motorcycle. Boisterous and loud, he called all of his male patients "buddy" and all of his female patients "hon." At times he pushed the operating room's decorum to its politically correct limits. Nevertheless, he was well liked, very bright, and extremely good at his job.

One dark October night Rich was called back to the hospital for an emergency. His prospective patient, an elderly man heading for the operating room for repair of a leaking aneurysm, needed an anesthesiologist quickly. Rich enjoyed torturing his bike's throttle even when he wasn't in much of a hurry, and he was soon rocketing down the glistening two-lane highway that connected his suburban home to the waiting ER. A frigid autumn rain had been falling for several hours, but Rich simply pulled his leather collar high around his neck and pushed on through the drizzle.

Halfway between home and the hospital, along a sinuous stretch of asphalt in the desolate Pennsylvania woodlands, Rich hit a sharp curve newly coated with damp leaves. As he leaned hard to take the turn, his front wheel hit the slippery vegetation and the bike slid out from beneath him. The machine toppled hard onto its left side and skittered across the blacktop with sparks flying, finally slamming into a low embankment. The impact threw Rich from his seat and he tumbled violently before coming to rest on the dank ground. Had he left the bike smoothly—like Hollywood stuntmen always do—he would have emerged unscathed, save for a few bruises. Swaddled in thick riding leathers and properly helmeted, Rich would have cursed himself, righted his dented vehicle, and continued on his way.

But his wingless flight wasn't smooth. As the crash tore his left hand from the handlebars, Rich's sleeve caught momentarily on the metal brake handle. It took just a fraction of a second for the arm to pull free, but that fraction would alter his life forever. He would relive that awful moment again and again in the months to come.

He remembers coming off the bike and, as he became airborne, feeling his left arm snap tautly like a thick piece of taffy before the handlebars twisted and freed him from the motorcycle. He also remembers the searing pain in his shoulder as the joint dislocated. But, most of all, he remembers a weird electric shock that zigzagged down his left arm and exited the tips of his fingers. After that odd sensation, there was nothing. All feeling in the arm vanished in an instant as if a fuse had blown somewhere in his body. He remembers thudding onto the ground and rolling countless times, his now-dead left arm flapping wildly like a stocking full of quarters and striking him repeatedly in the face and chest. His tumbling ended in a patch of icy mud at the foot of a large tree.

After catching his breath, Rich struggled to his feet and limped to his fallen bike, its rear wheel still angrily churning the chill night air. His left arm dangled flaccidly at his side, devoid of all movement and sensation, the hand rotated at a bizarre angle. The shoulder ached but the pain, surprisingly enough, quickly faded and no longer seemed bad at all…a temporary situation to be sure. With his good right arm, he shut down the engine and fished his portable phone from the bike's rear compartment. Ever the good physician, Rich first phoned the ER and told them to call his backup so that his erstwhile patient would not suffer from this night's folly. He then called the paramedics for himself and collapsed backward onto the deserted roadside.

As he waited for help to arrive, Rich nervously explored his injured arm. He found a strong radial pulse at the wrist; the accident had not harmed the arm's circulation. Grabbing the numb fingers, he lifted the limb, then let it fall clumsily to the ground. How heavy it felt, like ten pounds of cold sausage. He next probed the shoulder; no feeling there, either, but the shoulder joint was definitely out of place.

He then became aware of a faint tingling in his left abdomen and leg. Rich brushed at himself, afraid that ants had crawled into his clothing as he lay sprawled on the cold earth—but the season for ants had ended long ago. Rich, the trained physician, now realized with horror what had happened. The force of the crash had not only dislocated the shoulder joint, but had also injured the thick nerves in his upper arm, a bundle known as the brachial plexus. Mountain climbers suffer similar injuries when they jam their ice picks into the ground to halt a sudden fall. The weight of the entire body suddenly tugging on the arm can stretch the nerves or even tear them apart.

Rich held out hope that his was just a stretching injury, that the nerves had been momentarily stunned and would recover in a few hours, or at worst a few days. The ghostly ants crawling with increasing ferocity over his trunk and leg told him otherwise. The left side of his spinal cord must have been damaged; nothing else could explain the sensations in his leg. Some of the nerves must have ripped out of the spinal cord, thought Rich grimly, pulling bits of the cord's substance with them.

As an anesthesiologist, Rich was in charge of his hospital's chronic pain management clinic and had seen several patients with brachial plexus injuries in the past three years. He knew such patients can have ceaseless pain; panic set in as he realized he was about to become one of them. His arm, now an insensate chunk of lumber attached to a deformed shoulder, started to crawl with ants as well—the first inklings of the phantom sensations that would later drive him to the brink of suicide. So soon after his injury and already his nervous system played tricks on him.

Rich was about to become a victim of anesthesia dolorosa, or painful numbness. Also called phantom pain or denervation pain, anesthesia dolorosa is pain in a part of the body that no longer has sensation at all—one of nature's cruelest paradoxes.

As an ambulance wailed in the distance, Rich the macho weight lifter sat down in the mud and began to cry.

⭐

At a George Carlin performance I attended many years ago, the comedian reminisced about his mother's simplistic view of trauma. Carlin joked that his mother believed that only two types of injuries could ever befall a human body: broken necks and poked-out eyes. The nature of the injury depended upon what you held in your hands when calamity struck. If you fell down empty-handed, you broke your neck; if you fell down while holding a pencil, you lost an eye. Nothing else was possible in his mother's world. As a child, said Carlin, he always had a pencil in his hand while running or climbing trees, figuring that he would rather risk an eye than wind up a quadriplegic.

Like Carlin's mother, most people today (fortunately) have never experienced the terrible spectrum of real human trauma. That wasn't always the case. Our ancestors commonly had first-hand experience with the myriad manners in which a body can be broken—war wounds, torture, tumbles down rough terrain, attacks by wild beasts, hunting accidents, farming mishaps.

While horrific injuries were once part of primitive humans' daily fare, they have now become relatively rare in industrialized countries. Wild beasts no longer roam about freely. We walk on paved sidewalks instead of climbing through hazardous wilderness; we toss prepackaged meat into shopping carts instead of thundering on horseback after angry buffalo. Farms and factories, once breeding grounds of limb-threatening mayhem, have become reasonably safe. Even the gore of warfare has been reduced for us to two-dimensional images in newspapers or on television. Automobiles do their share to shred the human form, that's true, but even bad traffic accidents—our most common form of modern trauma—will affect few of us directly.

What little the average person knows about trauma is learned in movie theaters. In Hollywood bodily harm is a quantum event: you either die quickly or recover completely. There is no middle ground. Movie stars occasionally wear a sling or bandage for a scene or two, and may even limp or grimace once in a while, but they are rarely maimed on-screen. In his third Rambo movie, Sylvester Stallone absorbs an AK-47 bullet to his right knee but manages to walk away with a handkerchief wrapped about his leg. In reality, this projectile would have torn off his leg. In the film *Forrest Gump*, a buttock wound becomes a comical affair. A real bullet targeted at the sciatic nerve in the buttock is no laughing matter and would have rendered Gump as disabled as his double-amputee friend, Lieutenant Dan.

Even fatal injuries are minimalized on the big screen. At the conclusion of *The Champ*, a boxer endures a lethal head pounding and dies in his locker room after the bout. He remains lucid long enough for tear-jerking good-byes, then slips into a peaceful repose looking more like sleep than death. I know from personal experience that death from brain pulping is a far uglier and more prolonged affair than this.

Some directors—Stanley Kubrick and Sam Peckinpah come to mind—take great pains to portray injuries realistically, but their work is often decried as "too violent." We still like to see a lot of trauma on the screen, but we prefer it sanitized. Real trauma cannot be pasteurized, unfortunately, and not even a Kubrick could fabricate the bodily mayhem I have seen with my own eyes. Although trauma is much less frequent for us than it was for Neanderthals, modern humans keep their trauma victims alive much longer, thus allowing them to suffer the consequences of bad woundings for a lifetime. For some victims, the consequences can seem worse than a quick death. Dr. Rich McKnight would become one such victim.

His motorcycle accident tore apart the nerves in Rich's left arm and left it devoid of any sensation. As far as Rich's brain was concerned, the arm might as well have stayed forever in a ditch by the side of the road. To see why this type of total nerve injury causes chronic pain, we need to have some basic understanding of how pain signals are transmitted within the nervous system.

In the days before fire trucks, we fought fires by forming "bucket brigades" between the blaze and the nearest body of water. A line of people passed buckets of water hand over hand until the last person tossed it upon the flames. The nervous system employs a similar "brigade" strategy for relaying sensations into the brain. Each sensation—pain, temperature sense, deep pressure, fine touch, hearing, vision, smell, balance—employs a unique brigade of nerve cells, or neurons, linked together to relay information from the sense organ (skin, tongue, eye, ear, nose) to our conscious brains.

The technical name for pain sensation is nociception (Latin

noceo, "hurt," and *capio,* "receive"). The nociceptive brigade begins with specialized nerve endings in the skin. When we prick a finger, these nerve endings emit a burst of chemical signals resembling the dots and dashes of Morse code. The signals travel up the arm along nerve fibers at a speed of about ten feet per second; thousands of these tiny fibers bound together constitute a single nerve. The arm has three nerves—the median, ulnar, and radial—which join to form the brachial plexus in the shoulder.

After reaching the brachial plexus, pain signals from the arm and hand enter little clumps of nervous tissue known as ganglia, which lie alongside the spinal vertebrae. The ganglia then relay pain signals into the spinal cord. Deep within the central spinal cord lie clusters of nociceptive neurons that process the pain messages before passing them up the spinal cord to the brain. These microscopic nociceptive neurons are the culprits in anesthesia dolorosa.

Why does the body use a brigade system to relay messages from nerve ending to nerve, nerve to plexus, plexus to ganglia, ganglia to spinal cord, and spinal cord to brain? Why not simply pass sensory messages from the skin directly to the brain? A single nerve fiber can be several feet in length, so it is technically possible to link the brain cells directly to the hands and feet, without the need for numerous "go-between" nerve cells. Why doesn't the body use a simpler anatomy?

The brain is like the CEO of a large corporation. Pain messages can't be relayed directly to the brain for the same reason that the lowest employees can't have direct access to their CEO. In a corporation with thousands of employees, the CEO would quickly be overwhelmed with trivial problems best left to underlings—for example, how many paper clips does accounting need this month—and would be rendered incapable of making large-scale decisions.

The ganglia and nociceptive neurons act like middle managers, screening out small and inconsequential pain messages before they enter our conscious minds. Like real middle managers, they are also given the authority to make simpler decisions on their own, without any guidance from a higher authority. For example, if the nociceptive neurons in the spine receive information suggesting that a limb is in immediate danger of injury, they can activate the muscles in that limb to remove it from danger without first asking the brain's permission. Movement of a limb directed by the spinal cord alone, with no input from the brain, is called a reflex. By taking quick action, the spinal nociceptive neurons can shave a few milliseconds off the response time in a dangerous situation, time that might prevent a life-threatening injury. In very large animals—whales and extinct dinosaurs come to mind—the time saved by bypassing the brain may amount to a full second or longer. (That may be one reason why stupendously long-necked animals, like the apatosaurus, had such minuscule brains—the head was so far away from the action that most decisions had to be made in the spinal cord.)

Touch a hot stove and your hand jerks away before you even feel the pain. Your spinal nociceptive neurons felt the heat before you did and took action; only later was "the boss," aka your brain, informed of the situation. The spinal nociceptive neurons and their fellow middle managers in the body's pain apparatus stay active continuously—not just in the rare "hot stove" situations. They process information and send out signals to the muscles all the time and without our knowledge. As I sit here typing this sentence, I occasionally shift in my chair or move my arm to take the pressure off one area of my skin or to relieve prolonged strain on one part of my spine. Otherwise, I would be at risk for pressure sores, damaged nerves, and herniated discs.

We are typically oblivious to these constant adjustments; they are made even as we sleep. Even though the pain pathways are always working, we do not feel pain all of the time thanks to the (normally) wise discretion of the nociceptive neurons.

What do spinal nociceptive neurons have to do with phantom pain? As it turns out, everything. Like all good middle managers, nociceptive neurons do not like the boss to know they are idle, even when they have nothing of substance to do. When the department isn't busy, a smart manager will keep filing reports and memos to the CEO to make it seem like something big is still going on. The same is true for nociceptive neurons. They must stay busy even when they have nothing to do. And that can have nasty consequences.

When the motorcycle tore the nerves in Rich's left arm, the spinal nociceptive neurons programmed to receive pain sensations from that arm were suddenly "downsized"; without incoming sensations to process, they now had nothing to do. In order to appear busy, however, these neurons often resort to making things up, passing bogus signals to the brain's pain centers. With time, they may even go overboard, relaying so much false information to the brain that the conscious mind perceives little except constant pain—in a limb that no longer has a sensory supply or may not exist at all. Consequently, an amputee may feel burning in a foot that was cut away years earlier. Hence the name "phantom"—this is pain in a dead part of the body, the pain of a ghost. The medical name for this condition is deafferentation pain, but I prefer the more descriptive names phantom pain and denervation pain, or the more melodious anesthesia dolorosa.

Pleasant sensations don't behave in the same way. Why not?

Why aren't we flooded with pleasurable sensations from a missing limb? Pleasure is a much more complicated cognitive process relative to pain. Bogus signals emanating from unemployed spinal neurons don't have the complexity to register in our minds as pleasant. Consider a television set after the cable goes out. Despite the lack of intelligent input, as long as the set is turned on it will display a picture and emit sound. Television hardware is stupid in that it neither knows nor cares whether the images and noises it produces make any sense to us. Deprived of complex signals, the television's output will be irritating white snow and a grating buzz—hardly the Movie of the Week.

The spinal cord, like a television set, contains sophisticated switching and signal-processing hardware capable of miraculous things, but it also turns very stupid when all meaningful input ceases. The false signals relayed by denervated spinal neurons is akin to static. This static is perceived in the brain as pain since it arises in the area of the spinal cord responsible for pain signaling. Unlike TV static, there isn't an "off" switch for anesthesia dolorosa.

Thus, in the absence of any sensation, the spinal cord will feed us static and we will interpret it as burning pain. That's how we've been designed. Pain becomes the "default mode" of the nervous system. Perhaps there's some deep metaphysical message in this phenomenon—nothingness equals pain, but that's best left to professional philosophers.

~

Immediately upon Rich's arrival in the ER, an orthopedic surgeon returned his arm to its socket—a largely cosmetic exercise given the limb's ultimate uselessness. Shortly after Rich was admitted to our trauma center, radiologists injected an iodine dye into the spinal fluid pathways encircling his spinal cord, a procedure known as a myelogram. A CT scan of his neck showed the dye leaking from the spinal canal into the deep tissues of his neck. This proved Rich's roadside diagnosis had been on target; his plexus had been wrenched from the spine, leaving gaping holes in the spinal canal that permitted spinal fluid to seep into the surrounding muscles.

In the ensuing months, Rich's once muscular arm evaporated, turning into a withered stick. Therapists tried to keep the arm supple by bending and massaging his stiffening joints and tweaking the deteriorating muscles with galvanic current—all futile efforts. With no muscles to help hold the arm in place, his damaged shoulder joint dislocated again and again, forcing the orthopedists to wire the joint into permanent immobility. The arm finally froze into a position typical of complete plexus injuries: the elbow and fingers rigidly straight, the shoulder externally rotated, and the hand contracted ninety degrees at the wrist. Because it makes patients look like a haughty waiter soliciting a clandestine bribe behind his back, this posture is sometimes called the "maître d's pose."

Worse than the loss of a functional arm was the pain—burning, incessant pain that made Rich want to cleave his limb away with a machete. Most victims of denervation pain describe phantom sensations as burning or hot, although some complain of a sharper, intermittent pain similar to random electric shocks. Rich could never put his pain into words. He said that the English language couldn't do justice to what he felt.

Phantom pain can occur any time that cutaneous nerves are damaged with resultant numbness, even if the damage has been done therapeutically, as in the case of the alcohol injections once used to treat tic douloureux pains of the face. These injections were abandoned because of the high incidence of later anesthesia dolorosa. Rich manifested a particularly violent form of denervation pain—that of brachial plexus destruction. In addition to brachial plexus pain and the phantom limb pain of amputees, two less dramatic forms of denervation pain occur commonly: postherpetic neuralgia and diabetic neuropathy.

Diabetic neuropathy results from injury to the small nerves supplying the skin of the lower legs. This damage, in turn, stems from the microscopic vascular disease frequently found in long-standing diabetics. The nerves quite simply die of oxygen starvation, leading to numbness and, consequently, to denervation pain. Diabetics complain of burning in their feet, the typical description of anesthesia dolorosa.

Postherpetic pain—chronic pain after a herpes infection of the skin—is somewhat more complicated. Herpes is not a single virus but an extended family of viruses including those that cause cold sores, genital herpes, infectious mononucleosis, chicken pox, and shingles. The last two afflictions—chicken pox and shingles—are the product of a single virus, herpes zoster, the virus responsible for most postherpetic neuralgia.

Although herpetic infections look like skin rashes, most herpes species aren't skin viruses but nerve viruses. Although a herpetic infection frequently begins in the skin, the viruses quickly migrate up the nerves and take up permanent residence in the spinal ganglia. There they may lie dormant forever or decide to take regular pilgrimages back to the skin and cause rashes again and again—hence the recurring bouts of facial and genital sores that can occur long after the primary infection has healed. The viruses aren't being nasty for the sake of being nasty; they have to resurface and shed themselves through weeping skin blisters to complete their reproductive cycle.

Shingles, a chest wall rash that afflicts mostly older adults and people with compromised immune systems, is nothing more than a localized recurrence of childhood chicken pox. But this is a pox with an attitude. During an attack of shingles, chest wall nerves can be severely damaged, even destroyed by reproducing viruses. For most people, this creates only a vague aching or itching at the site of the healed rash. For others, the damage may set off phantom pains so severe that they are mistaken for heart attacks, gallbladder spasms, blood clots to the lungs, even cancer.

Many physicians don't realize that postherpetic neuralgia is a form of anesthesia dolorosa. They treat it with nerve blocks, skin creams, and other localized therapies that prove useless or may make matters worse. John D., a seventy-five-year-old retired steelworker and past patient of mine, is a case in point.

John has lymphoma. He responded well to chemotherapy and his prognosis is good, but after his final chemotherapy treatment he developed a severe case of shingles covering his entire left chest below the nipple. Aggressive use of antiviral drugs shortened the acute infection and his lesions soon scabbed over and healed. After several months his slight chest wall numbness gradually gave way to searing pain. Narcotics provided scant relief and his oncologist sent him to our pain clinic; once there, an anesthesiologist repeatedly injected the spinal nerves with local anesthetic. This helped a bit and so John was referred to a thoracic surgeon, who promptly cut the nerves.

To John's dismay, cutting his nerves only poured fuel on the flames that burned in his chest. Instead of helping him, nerve destruction made him worse. By the time I saw him, he was so saturated with sedatives and painkillers that he could barely speak. I referred him to the pain surgeon who would eventually operate upon Rich McKnight. He was cured, but more about that later.

We now know that anesthesia dolorosa doesn't originate in the skin or nerves but in the miscreant nociceptive neurons deep within the gelatinous substance of the spinal cord. Damage to peripheral skin nerves causes anesthesia dolorosa in the first place; creating more nerve damage to treat the pain only risks making it worse. Why do temporary nerve blocks help? No one knows. The answer may lie in the brain's endorphin system, which acts as a source of natural morphine.

Since the problem lies in the spinal cord, the cure for anesthesia dolorosa must be found there as well. But the spinal cord is a therapeutic no-man's-land, a treacherous minefield where one surgical misstep can yield disaster. Nevertheless, clinicians must obey Sutton's rule, named for the notorious bandit Willie Sutton. When asked why he robbed banks, Sutton answered simply, "Because that's where they keep the money." Sutton's rule of medicine states that the doctor, like a bank robber, must go to where the money is, regardless of how dangerous or fortified the vault may be. In anesthesia dolorosa, the money lies buried in the nociceptive neurons, deep within the most fragile and unforgiving anatomy that we possess.

As the first anniversary of his accident came and went, Rich found himself sinking further into depression. He couldn't work, nor could he exercise. He tried to lift weights again but his heart simply wasn't in it. He once believed that the hours he spent run-

ning and lifting were for his health and well-being, but he now realized that his workouts served only his vanity. Now that his left
arm looked like the gnarled branch of a dead tree, preserving his
precious body image didn't seem worth the effort anymore.

He had been on and off narcotics ever since the accident,
everything from small-time pills to long-acting morphine preparations and topical fentanyl patches. Drugs helped some, but they
never worked all that well. But then, drugs are for pain, and the
incessant heat in his arm...well, it was awful but it didn't seem
like pain. It was just there all of the time. When he ate, when he
showered, when he watched television, even when he got up in
the night to go to the bathroom—there it was. Day in and day out,
his dead fingers howled like unhappy ghosts in the cemetery of
his arm. You're gone, he would tell his hand, useless and gone,
leave me in peace.

Narcotics made him dreamy and made things more bearable
at times, but he knew this wasn't a healthy way to deal with his
problem. Like drinking to ease the grief of losing a loved one,
taking narcotics for chronic pain only distracts; it can't cure. Real
healing takes something more. That's what he used to tell his own
pain patients. If only he could believe it himself.

Rich's depression—like depression in any chronic pain patient—derived not only from his physical pain, but from his feelings of hopelessness. The fear of never being out of pain, of
never being whole again, haunts chronic pain sufferers and forces
them to contemplate suicide or to seek out any therapy, no matter how expensive and bizarre. Rich ate large doses of vitamin E,
rubbed herbal preparations on his arm, and put copper bracelets
on his wrists. He went to a chiropractor, an acupuncturist, even a
faith healer (under assumed names, of course).

In a fit of anger, he stormed into the office of an orthopedic surgeon and demanded that his arm be amputated. The surgeon's gentle reminder that his pain wasn't in the arm but in Rich's central nervous system didn't dissuade him. "The dumb thing just gets in the way; I'm better off without it," Rich complained. The surgeon appeased him and scheduled an amputation for the following month, but Rich backed out, as the surgeon knew he would. Withered though it was, it was still his arm, the arm of his youth, an arm that once sported the best baseball mitt his allowance money could buy. He never could bring himself to toss that mitt away, and now he wouldn't toss his arm away, either. Yes, the mitt and the arm were now relics, useless mementos of happier times. Such mementos are not easily discarded.

One morning, when he felt he no longer could face another day, Rich drove to a gas station and filled his tank in the grim expectation of shutting himself in his garage and letting carbon monoxide take care of the situation once and for all. As he drove into the garage and closed the door behind him, he abruptly shut down the engine and pounded his fist on the steering wheel. He wouldn't give up without trying the one procedure that he knew might help but that terrified him nonetheless: DREZ lesioning. For two months he had carried in his wallet the phone number of the local neurosurgeon specializing in the operation. Rich went upstairs, unfolded the wrinkled notepaper, and dialed the number. He would have to travel to another city for an appointment, but that wouldn't be a problem.

After all, he had just filled his gas tank.

✥

The nociceptive neurons lie in an area of the spinal cord known as the dorsal root entry zone: DREZ. Without going into the stupefying details, the DREZ lies in the backward-facing part of the spinal cord, just deep to the region where the spinal roots exit. (The word *dorsal* comes from the Latin *dorsum,* meaning "back"—think of the dorsal fin of a shark or dolphin.)

In the 1970s renowned pain surgeon Blaine Nashold of Duke University found that opening the spine and destroying the nociceptive neurons with a heated probe shallowly inserted into the DREZ would relieve the pain of anesthesia dolorosa in selected patients. The operation came to be known as DREZ lesioning, or, more simply, as the DREZ operation. The theory behind the DREZ operation is quite simple: Since anesthesia dolorosa arises from hallucinating nociceptive neurons in the spinal cord, the surgeon must enter the spinal cord and destroy those neurons. Those crazy middle managers must be silenced.

Many patients with brachial plexus injuries never get anesthesia dolorosa. When the nerves of these patients are ripped from the spinal cord by excessive traction on the arm, the nociceptive neurons are pulled out of the spinal cord along with them. In effect, these patients undergo DREZ lesioning at the time of their accidents. Rich had some nerves pulled out of the cord, while others tore in the shoulder, leaving the spinal nociceptive neurons unscathed. It was these undamaged neurons that caused him to teeter on the brink of self-destruction. Nashold felt that he could eliminate phantom arm pains in patients like Rich by surgically destroying any nociceptive cells that survived the accident intact.

DREZ lesioning has a dark side. The surgeon must create a controlled injury to the spinal cord using either heat (a thermal probe) or extreme cold (a cryoprobe). In either case, there is no way to limit precisely how much of the cord will be damaged. Too small a lesion and the operation will fail. Too big a lesion and the motor pathways to the arms, legs, or bladder could be affected, causing paralysis or incontinence. During a DREZ operation, the surgeon is tossing a hand grenade into the spinal cord and hoping the explosion kills all the bad guys and none of the good guys. Amazingly enough, that's what almost always happens. Almost always, but not always.

For Rich, the thought of ending up a paraplegic reduced to having a single functioning limb terrified him so much that he refused to consider the procedure even though he had seen it work wonders in his own patients. But now, it was either DREZ lesioning or suicide. There was no longer any third option.

Sixteen months after his accident, Rich underwent DREZ lesioning. We exposed his cervical spinal cord and placed a dozen thermal lesions in the DREZ along the left border of his spinal cord. Under the operating microscope, the damage wrought on that terrible autumn night now loomed large. Divots and scar tissue marred the normally marble-smooth surface of Rich's spinal cord. A few severed nerves, shriveled and stained a rusty brown from old hemorrhage, floated in the pulsating spinal fluid like fronds of dead seaweed.

When I open someone up and peer at an injury that is months or years old, I feel like an oceanographer seeing a lost shipwreck for the first time. I can't help but imagine how the ruined organ appeared in its pristine state; I also instinctively see in my mind's eye the events that rendered this marvelous machinery useless and decrepit. I'm certain that shipwreck explorers are likewise haunted by visions of water pouring through damaged hulls and the death howls of sailors long gone. For me, seeing a withered, lifeless nerve torn apart by trauma is like seeing a child's doll lying on the bottom of the sea. It gives me a hollow feeling, a feeling of something wonderful that has been lost, never to be regained.

Postoperatively, Rich's left foot was weak for several days, the temporary result of spinal cord swelling. Some of the good guys in his spinal cord had been knocked down by our grenades, but they soon righted themselves and went back to work. His weakness soon faded. Otherwise, he suffered no ill effects. The pain vanished, the screaming ghosts of his departed hand exorcised forever. The coagulating heat of the DREZ probe had driven away the eternal burning in his arm. Fire conquering fire.

Rich quit anesthesia. Even without his pain, he could no longer perform his job to the level to which he had become accustomed. Supported by his disability income, he entered a physical medicine residency and became a rehabilitation specialist. His depression cleared and he later remarried.

He kept the baseball mitt...but sold the motorcycle.

➤

DREZ lesioning has been used successfully for brachial plexus avulsion injuries, phantom limb pain, postherpetic neuralgia, even facial pain syndromes. My patient John, the lymphoma survivor with postshingles chest pain, was similarly cured by DREZ lesioning. Although—theoretically, anyway—the DREZ operation should help diabetic neuropathy as well, DREZ lesioning for that devilish condition is technically more challenging and rarely worth the effort. Fortunately, diabetic neuropathy tends not to reach the intensity of brachial plexus pain and post-herpetic neuralgia. Moreover, newer drugs such as Neurontin have proven effective in managing the burning feet of diabetics, making surgery needless.

No pain procedure works for everyone and DREZ lesioning can fail. In some cases, the operation works initially, but a new kind of pain returns months or years postoperatively. This post-DREZ pain may be due to neuronal hallucinations farther upstream in the nociceptive brigade, perhaps in the brain itself. Like other destructive procedures, DREZ lesioning can work miracles but also carries some risk of relocating the nervous system's dysfunction elsewhere and creating an even more troublesome pain syndrome months or years later. Although surgeons can chase phantom pain into the brain, the risks of therapeutic lesioning there are greater and the results less satisfactory.

Phantom sensations occur in other sensory systems as well. For example, a disturbing ringing in the ears known as tinnitus often accompanies hearing loss. This ringing, which is actually more like a loud whining, comes from nerve cells feeding static to the hearing centers of the brain for lack of anything better to do, just as anesthesia dolorosa comes from spinal neurons feeding static to the brain's pain centers. Tinnitus also shares with phantom pain a resistance to easy treatment.

Years ago I heard a story, perhaps apocryphal but illustrative nonetheless, about an outside electrical contractor who had been summoned to my father's factory, where a large rolling mill had suddenly refused to work. The electrician quickly replaced one of the machine's numerous circuit boards and the mill immediately sprang to life. He presented his bill: five hundred dollars for labor.

"Five hundred dollars to replace a circuit board in five minutes?" asked an angry superintendent.

"No," the electrician replied, "ten dollars to replace the board, four hundred and ninety dollars for knowing which board to replace."

In pain surgery, too, the skill lies not only in fixing the electrical flaw, but knowing where to find it. Thanks to pioneers like Nashold, we now have the tools to do just that.

3   "TIC-DOLLY-ROW"

It's a kind of tic-dolly-row they say—worse nor a toothache. Well, well; I don't know what it is, but the Lord keep me from catching it...

—Herman Melville, *Moby Dick*

One bright and colorful autumn day, Mildred first noticed the vague itching on the right side of her nose. She was raking the yard and blamed the chilly breeze that blew across her face. But the itch didn't go away when she went indoors. In fact, it persisted for weeks, making her paw at her cheek incessantly like a cat grooming its face. One day shortly after Thanksgiving, she reached up to swipe at the itch as she had done a thousand times before and the pain came, a blazing heat that flared across her cheek and burrowed deep into her nostril and empty gums. Seventy-three years old, Mildred had lost her own teeth years ago, but this pain was worse than any toothache she had ever known. The pain made her shriek, a sound that hadn't crossed her lips since Eisenhower was president, when she last gave birth. Her legs buckled for an instant, but she recovered quickly and managed not to fall over.

Then, as quickly as it had come, the pain ceased. She glanced down at her hand, expecting to see blood. She must have scratched herself badly with a fingernail, she thought, but there wasn't any bleeding. What had happened? She touched her cheek again and the pain returned, somewhat less intense but still dreadful. After a few timorous taps on her sore cheek, the paroxysms finally ended, leaving Mildred worried and perplexed. What did this all mean? Perhaps nothing. She forgot about it until the next day.

Mildred awoke the following morning and her first act of the new day, as it had been for over fifty years, was to reach for her eyeglasses. But as she slid the frames onto her face, the pain returned with a fury. Alarmed, she removed them quickly, then tried again. After repeated trials she finally managed to keep them on, but from then on any sudden movement of her head would jar the glasses slightly and bring the iron spikes driving deep into her face once more. The threat of pain forced her to move slowly and gingerly, as though she were walking on thin ice or balancing an invisible encyclopedia on her head.

More unpleasant surprises awaited her. She couldn't tolerate her upper denture plate at all, and the simple act of drinking something a little too hot or too cold proved unbearable. Mildred thought she had been rid of these sensations after her hopelessly decayed teeth had been removed. She knew that something would have to be done, else she would spend her remaining years drinking lukewarm coffee and gumming oatmeal.

She went to her dentist. He didn't find anything wrong but gave Mildred a gel to rub on her gums and sent her to see her family doctor. The family doctor couldn't find anything wrong, either, so she referred Mildred to an oral surgeon, who also gave her a clean bill of health—but suggested she consult a sinus surgeon just to be on the safe side. The sinus surgeon took a few X rays and gave her a good once-over before pronouncing her fit and healthy. But Mildred wasn't healthy. Three months had passed since the pains came, and she had dropped twenty pounds.

Now when Mildred looked in a mirror, she no longer saw a robust widow enjoying her senior years but an impostor: a gaunt, toothless hag with her glasses bent away from her face to keep the pain at bay, someone who looked like one of the pitiful old women who inhabited her late husband's nursing home.

She soon couldn't even speak without contorting her mouth in anguished knots. She avoided friends and family, even her beloved grandchildren, so that she wouldn't have to talk at all. The few people she was forced to interact with—delivery boys, meter readers—had to make do with her limited repertoire of irritated hand gestures. A once full and vigorous life began to contract and shrivel into a life confined to four walls, the precious time wasted in anxious anticipation of the next wave of pain.

Going outside in the blowing air was risky so she never ventured beyond her front door unless absolutely necessary. Summer arrived, but Mildred dared not turn on the air conditioner or (heaven forbid!) sit in front of a fan for fear of turning her face into a seething cauldron. Sleeping became a special challenge; the pain stalked her in the night, startling her out of a deep sleep like a mischievous child. As weeks turned into months, Mildred descended into the world of chronic pain. Her affliction now dictated every aspect of her life: where she could go, what she could eat, whom she could see, what she could do, even how she could sleep. Her identity merged with her suffering, and Mildred soon become one with her facial pain. She had become a victim of Melville's "tic-dolly-row."

⤙

The *Iliad*'s Helen of Troy possessed a face so beautiful that it was said to have launched a thousand ships. The Phantom of the Opera, on the other hand, possessed a countenance so vile that it drove him into permanent exile within the dank bowels of the Paris Opera House. Homer's heroic Helen and Leroux's tragic Phantom, although fictional extremes, are no different from the rest of us—our faces shape our lives. The human face does double duty, serving as both passport to the outside world and window to our souls. A mother's face is the first image her infant recognizes, and children learn to read emotion on the faces of others as they quickly assimilate the spoken word.

Physiognomy—the "science" of predicting a person's intelligence, personality, even moral character, using precise measurements of facial anatomy—was widely accepted in the last century, particularly in Europe. Criminal defendants could be convicted simply because they had "criminal" faces. Sir Arthur Conan Doyle believed strongly in physiognomy, and his Sherlock Holmes mysteries contain frequent references to the "high brow" of the intellectual and the "narrow eyes" of the common thief. Oscar Wilde's Dorian Gray delays, but cannot prevent, the ultimate facial corruption caused by the progressive degeneracy of his character. And the Phantom's twisted visage—was it an accident of birth or the outward manifestation of his tortured soul?

Of course, we now consider physiognomy more of a

pseudoscience than a true science, but its core hypothesis—that a person's fundamental essence is somehow reflected in craniofacial anatomy—contains some kernel of truth. Although no one undergoes the transformation of Dorian Gray, any face over time will reveal something of the life and character of the person behind it. As George Orwell noted with his typical cynicism, "At fifty, everyone has the face he deserves."

Ancient philosophers considered the heart to be the seat of the soul; this idea gave way to the more intuitive notion that humanity emanates from the head, not the chest. The head houses the brain and four of the five major senses: vision, hearing, taste, and smell. In mammals, the face also serves as a major organ for fine touch and pain discrimination as well. Thus, the lion's share of our sensory input comes from sense organs located mere inches from the brain. In a literal sense, we live in our heads; we *are* our heads. Actor Christopher Reeve no longer feels or controls any part of his body below his upper neck, yet the human spark that defines him as a person survived his accident undamaged.

The amount of brain dedicated to processing sensory information arising in the scalp, face, and mouth is larger than that dedicated to sensations coming from the rest of the body combined (save for the hands). This heightened sensitivity makes the head and face fertile ground for a number of cruel pain syndromes.

As Mildred discovered, there is something devilish about pains arising in the face and head. They strike us at the geometric center of our beings. Our consciousness resides, after all, within the confines of our skulls. A leg pain arrives in our consciousness telegraphed from some friendly but vaguely distant land, while the severe headache or face pain barges into the mind's home like an unsavory intruder. When our head or face hurts, *we* hurt, and in a very profound way.

The fiendishness doesn't end there. Cranial pain syndromes border on the surreal. Even as they torment victims with years of blinding pain, they leave little or no trace of pathology behind in their wake, making their victims appear healthy and without physical evidence of illness. These are stealth diseases gliding beneath the radar of our medical technology, clinical torturers without portfolios.

Cancer pain is terrible, but we can understand how something that erodes our bones and devours our nerves will be painful. Cancer is a destructive disease, and such diseases cause pain. We may not agree with cancer's agenda, but at least it possesses one. The same goes for rheumatoid arthritis; rheumatoid joints look inflamed, swollen, and misshapen—the joints make no secret of their need to hurt, and a terrible pathology is obviously to blame. But where, or what, is the disease in migraine sufferers? Or in patients troubled by neuralgias of the face or throat? The diseases giving rise to these pains may be difficult or impossible to detect, or may be so subtle—a brain artery in the wrong place, a simple food allergy, a few misaligned teeth—as to seem trivial.

People with cranial pain syndromes often look quite robust, a facade that masks their terrible afflictions. A healthy appearance can worsen the psychological trauma of pain; family, friends, even medical professionals, may have difficulty believing anything is seriously wrong, and may even accuse the patient of exaggerating or malingering. A man with metastatic prostate cancer garners sympathy while a coworker who calls off because of a migraine does not, even though migraine pain can be as incapacitating as cancer pain at times.

I must confess here that I have a personal interest in face pain.

As a lifelong migraine sufferer, I am well acquainted with the nastiness of head pain. Moreover, I did my neurosurgical training in one of the world's foremost centers for the surgical treatment of facial pain disorders, where I was weaned professionally on a steady diet of facial pain. It was there that I met Mildred...and hundreds more like her.

⇒

Pain syndromes of the head and face are grouped in a common category of craniofacial pain disorders known as cephalgias, from the Greek *kephalos* (head) and *algos* (pain). The scalp and face share a common sensory pathway, so that pain in one area of the head often radiates to other areas. Head pains like migraine can affect the cheeks, nose, and eyes; facial pain syndromes may affect the scalp. Although we commonly think of the face as a patch of skin extending from cheek to cheek horizontally and from chin to hairline vertically, the "anatomic" face also includes the teeth, the ears, most of the scalp, and, amazingly enough, the leathery inner lining of the skull.

These structures all transmit touch and pain sensations to the brain through two trigeminal nerves, one for the right side of the head and one for the left. Each trigeminal nerve, about the diameter of a child's crayon, lies just deep to the cheekbone. The nerve derives its name from the Greek word *trigeminos*, meaning "three origins," a reference to the nerve's three facial branches. The first branch carries sensations from the scalp, eyes, and forehead; the second, from the cheeks, nose, upper lip, and upper teeth; the third, from the jaw, tongue, lower lip, and lower teeth.

The medical name for tic douloureux is trigeminal neuralgia, or TN as it's commonly abbreviated. The word *neuralgia* literally means "nerve pain" and TN results from disease within the trigeminal nerve itself. Although the face and teeth hurt terribly, there is no pathology there; unfortunately, this doesn't stop dentists from pulling healthy teeth, and ear, nose, and, throat surgeons from cleaning out healthy sinuses in vain attempts to cure the disorder.

TN patients rarely have constant pain, but instead suffer lightninglike bursts of facial or oral pain that last for several seconds and then vanish. The word typically used to describe these volleys of pain is *lancinating*, from the Latin *lancinatus*, meaning "to rend or rip." This word says a lot about the character of TN pain, which has been likened to having one's face shredded. TN produces paroxysms of searing, shocklike pain along one or more of the three trigeminal branches. Most patients experience only pain in the cheeks, jaw, or lower teeth. Pains affecting the scalp, eyes, or entire face are quite rare. The flashes of TN pain are brief but terrifying, frequently causing the patient to wince after each paroxysm. This staccato wincing caused early observers to consider TN a tic, or facial spasm, hence the older name tic douloureux, or painful tic.

Victims compare their TN paroxysms to the salvos of nerve pain that result when a dentist's drill strikes too deeply. The salvos may fire off sporadically or, more commonly, are triggered by touching the affected area. Cold air blowing against the face, the acts of teeth brushing or simple chewing can also bring on the pain.

John Locke gave the first clear description of TN in 1677, when he was called to see the wife of the English ambassador to France:

*On Thursday night last, I was sent for to my Lady
Ambassadrice, whom I found in a fit of such violent and exquisite
torment...as you would expect from one upon the rack.... When
the fit came, there was, to use my Lady's own expression of it, as
it were a flash of fire all of a sudden shot into all those parts....
Speaking was apt to put her into these fits; sometimes opening her
mouth to take anything, or touching her gums....*

Women are more affected than men by a ratio of two to one, and more than 70 percent of victims are over fifty years old when the disease first strikes. Although it may onset following a dental procedure (for as yet unknown reasons) or may occur in association with multiple sclerosis, TN usually arises spontaneously and with no known inciting event or concurrent disease.

The pain of TN resembles the erratic dripping of Chinese water torture; both produce random discomfort more subtle and devious than constant pain. We can sometimes adapt to constant pain, but TN's sporadic jolts keep its victims off balance. Patients might go hours, even a few days or weeks without feeling the shocks, but the paroxysms always return. Mildred later told me that her pain-free episodes were often the hardest part of the disease to bear because they were filled only by the dreadful expectation of the inevitable.

The cruelty of water torture lies in its unpredictability. If victims could anticipate each drop of water, they would soon block out the sensation. The same is true of TN. The paroxysms have no rhythm, coming in chaotic bursts that prevent TN patients from habituating to the pain. TN sufferers spend much of

---

* Stookey, B., and J. Ransohoff, J. *Trigeminal Neuralgia: Its History and Treatment* (Springfield, Ill.: Charles C. Thomas, 1959).

their time guessing when the next droplet of pain will splash on their faces, never sure when it will come or what might set it off. Like Christ in Gethsemane, they dread the certainty of future pain as much as the pain itself. Like an expert torturer, TN breaks the spirit and establishes itself as master.

Mildred was stronger than most patients I had seen. She wasn't like the broken ones who dragged spouses and children into their quicksands of pain. I have witnessed husbands quitting their jobs to make new careers out of their wives' TN, and wives spoon-feeding their husbands before trundling them from specialist to specialist like pampered royalty. Even the strongest edifices of human dignity can become cracked and eroded by the daily onslaught of unbearable pain. Mildred's dignity hadn't tumbled down, not yet, and she decided to take matters into her own hands.

Dissatisfied with the nonanswers provided by her previous physicians and dentists, she became an aggressive patient and sought out the opinion of an excellent neurologist, who immediately recognized her problem as TN. He started her on phenytoin, a drug normally used to control epileptic seizures but with proven benefit in reducing the pains of TN. This helped her a little, but not much. He then switched her to carbamazine, another antiseizure medication—more effective but somewhat riskier than phenytoin—and Mildred soon thought she had been cured. Her pains ceased for almost six months. She regained her lost weight, repaired her bent glasses, and had her dentures refitted.

Unfortunately, routine blood tests showed that her liver enzymes were rising, an early sign that the miraculous carbamazine was inflicting subtle but dangerous liver damage, a side effect of the drug in elderly patients taking the large doses needed to control TN. Mildred's TN required a carbamazine dose almost twice that needed to stop epilepsy. Mildred's neurologist reduced the dosage, but the enzyme levels continued to rise. Even worse, she began experiencing those old familiar twinges again as the chemical bonds restraining the beast were loosened and the disease struggled to wrench free. Despite the pain, the drug had to be stopped before her liver damage became irreversible. Quickly, the beast broke loose once more.

Mildred flew into a blind panic. After the carbamazine was stopped, the stabbing pains came more frequently than ever, as if the disease had been angered by her attempts to slay it and sought revenge. Her neurologist tried baclofen, another good TN drug, but that did little except make her drowsy and confused. She spent her nights crying and contemplating suicide. The act of sobbing worsened her paroxysms, so sensitive was her cheek now that even tears running down it brought on the pain. Like an abusive parent, the illness beat her harder for crying.

She kept her wits until her neurologist tried her on morphine elixir. When that failed she started to come unglued. If morphine, the most potent and addictive of pain medications, didn't work, what would? Mildred now faced the hell feared by Bertrand Russell—she stood on the edge of the ferocious abyss, looking down at a life of pain without end. Her affliction seemed bullet proof; nothing could touch it. The TN didn't even have the common courtesy of killing her. Even cancer was kinder in that regard. Hers wasn't a sickness, after all, just pain, pure and senseless pain. Doctors told her she was healthy, but her health seemed like a liability to Mildred now, something to keep her alive longer. Her daughter, afraid that Mildred teetered on the brink of disaster, brought her to the university hospital where I was training in neurosurgery. It was time for more drastic measures—brain surgery.

⟡

Nerves may look like simple wires, but even the tiniest one is a complex cable containing many thousands of different nerve fibers. A nerve fiber is a fingerlike extension, or axon, extruded by the body of a single nerve cell, and may range from a few inches to a few feet in length. There are two basic categories of fibers: motor fibers, which transmit impulses from the nervous system to the muscles of the body; and sensory fibers, which carry impulses from the body back to the nervous system.

In nerves carrying skin sensation, like the trigeminal nerve, sensory nerve fibers can be further divided into two classes: fibers carrying touch sensation and fibers carrying pain sensations. This is a point of inestimable importance in pain therapeutics: the sensations of touch and pain travel separate roads on their journey to the brain.

When a noise becomes too loud, it turns painful; likewise, an excessively bright light will hurt our eyes. In these instances, pain represents the extreme limit of normal sound or light sensation. However, in the skin, pain isn't an excess of touch but a completely different sensation altogether, possessing its own hardware in the nervous system. By targeting this pain hardware only, it's theoretically possible for clinicians, surgeons in particular, to eliminate pain sensation in the skin without rendering the skin numb to touch.

The pain fibers are, from an evolutionary point of view, the oldest and most primitive fibers in the nervous system, evidence of the primordial role that aversive reflexes play in animals. Pain fibers are little more than bare wires, with almost no surrounding "insulation" to protect them. The touch fibers, in contrast, wear a thick insulating coat of myelin, an ivory-colored fat that gives the white matter of the brain its distinctive hue. Myelin—from the Greek word *myelos,* meaning "marrow" (myelin is to nerve what marrow is to bone)—electrically isolates the touch fibers from the exposed pain fibers and prevents "cross-talk" between touch and pain pathways. Any breaks in this insulation will create short circuits between the two pathways, enabling pain sensations to enter touch pathways and vice versa.

In TN patients, myelin is damaged or missing in the trigeminal nerve, usually near the nerve's entry point into the brain; this myelin loss allows touch and pain sensations arising in the facial skin to become scrambled, leading to confusion in upstream sensory centers within the higher brain. When something touches the facial skin, nerve signals start out in the appropriate touch fibers but end up jumping over to pain fibers in the damaged area of the trigeminal nerve, entering the conscious brain in the wrong place and making the lightest touch feel like burning pain. The damage to the trigeminal's myelin may be minute—a tiny injury barely a fraction of an inch in size is sufficient to cause the disease. Here is the surreal nature of facial pain: people can be driven to suicide by pain simply because they are missing a piece of nerve fat the size of a flea.

Antiepileptic drugs like carbamazine and phenytoin prevent seizures by halting the spread of abnormal electrical activity in the brain. Their ability to limit "short-circuiting" in the brain's wiring probably explains their effectiveness in treating TN and other forms of nerve pain. They can produce dramatic results but cause such severe side effects (liver injury, rashes, dizziness, anemia) that they can rarely be employed to control TN for a lifetime. Surgery becomes the next, and only, alternative.

What causes the myelin damage leading to TN? In some cases, the trigeminal damage is just a small part of a larger-scale myelin deterioration taking place throughout the central nervous system: multiple sclerosis. But MS causes only about 1 or 2 percent of all TN cases in the general population. In another handful of TN cases, the nerve is damaged by tumors, vascular lesions (like aneurysms), or deformities at the base of the skull where the nerve penetrates the bone on its way to the brain. What causes the other 90 percent of TN cases?

Something rather odd, as it turns out. In the 1930s legendary Baltimore neurosurgeon Walter Dandy noted that the trigeminal nerves of TN patients were frequently compressed by the arteries at the base of the brain. As we age, atherosclerosis causes our brain arteries to elongate and become looped and coiled upon themselves, forming redundant, pulsating spirals. Further complicating matters, the aging brain begins to sag (like everything else in our aging bodies), pulling the trigeminal nerves downward against the hardening arteries at the base of the skull. Dandy theorized that TN could be caused by a coiled artery accidentally wedging itself against the trigeminal nerve. The incessant pounding of arterial blood within an aging, calcified artery would eventually damage the nerve's myelin, short-circuiting touch and pain pathways and giving rise to TN.

His theory made sense. It explained why TN occurs more frequently in older patients, who have harder and more tortuous arteries (and sagging brains). It also explained why TN pain prefers the lower part of the face: the lower branches of the nerve turn out to be the most vulnerable to arterial compression. To prove his theory, Dandy published illustrations of TN patients' trigeminal nerves with deep grooves carved into them by way-ward arteries.

In Dandy's model, TN becomes just another painful manifes-tation of the degenerative process, the result of hardening arter-ies banging against lax brain structures. Our arteries become like rats in the brain's basement, slowly gnawing at the wiring until some electrical disaster occurs. For diseases of aging, like TN, we can't look to "natural" solutions. Nature saw no need to provide us with any since TN affects mostly people beyond their "natu-ral" life spans. Except for the last half a century (and even then, only in developed nations), human life expectancy was typically below forty years. Maladies such as cancer, heart disease, arthri-tis, and TN are modern curses, targeting the burgeoning popula-tions of elderly who have been shielded by technology from the ravages of natural selection. As such, there are no simple lifestyle changes or herbal remedies that will ameliorate TN. More often than not, patients require surgical intervention.

Moving the offending arteries away from the nerve would seem the obvious surgical solution, but, curiously, Dandy never tried it, preferring instead to cut part of the nerve at the base of the brain. It was during these nerve-cutting operations that Dandy made the seminal observations leading to his vascular compression model of TN's causation, yet these observations didn't sway his belief in nerve sectioning. Dandy was an extra-ordinarily brilliant man—one of the founding fathers of modern brain surgery—but his thinking was hamstrung by the paradigm governing surgical pain therapy in his era—namely, if a nerve causes pain, destroy it. Prior to the 1950s no adequate drug ther-

apy of TN existed, and so all TN therapies were surgical therapies. And all surgical therapies required destruction (ablation) of
the main nerve or one of its three facial branches. As pioneering
surgeon Frank Hartley wrote in 1892: "We can not be reasonably
certain of a good prognosis until all branches...in which pain is
present are cut."

At the turn of the century, the typical TN surgery consisted
of isolating one of the three trigeminal branches in the face (or
the main trunk of the nerve just under the temporal lobe of the
brain) and crushing or cutting it or, even grislier, winding it up on
a piece of metal like so much living spaghetti and yanking it out.
What an atrocious ordeal this must have been in the preanesthesia era, especially for TN patients barely able to tolerate the wind
against their exposed cheeks.

In the early part of this century, needle procedures for the
cure of TN were introduced. In these procedures, the surgeon
advances a long needle through the cheekbone into the base of
the skull, then destroys the main trunk of nerve either by injecting absolute alcohol through the needle or by heating the needle
with an electric current. Although useful, these so-called ablative
procedures had a dark side. While they frequently (but not uni-
versally) eliminated the paroxysms of TN, needle ablations also
resulted in dense facial numbness that, over time, could prove
more of a problem than the original TN. If the eye became anesthetic, not an uncommon complication, patients had a high like-
lihood of corneal scarring and eventual blindness, and a small
number of patients developed that virulent pain syndrome experienced by Rich McKnight: anesthesia dolorosa, the "painful
numbness."

Although they were more tolerable than tearing out the
nerve, needle procedures weren't exactly a picnic. In the early

days of my training, we still commonly tried heating the nerve using a needle electrode. Twenty years have passed and I can still hear the patients screaming. We would stuff blankets around the doors to muffle their anguished cries so that patients in other operating rooms wouldn't be disturbed. Inflicting this type of pain wasn't easy on the surgeon either, and we used to joke grimly that the needle operation was little more than two terrified people separated by an electrode.

Dandy advocated opening the skull, moving aside the brain tissue covering the nerve, and *partially* cutting the nerve near its entry point into the brain stem located at the top of the spinal cord; it was a far riskier procedure than complete needle destruction because it required full-blown brain surgery. Nevertheless, Dandy believed that this procedure carried a lower risk of total facial numbness and subsequent anesthesia dolorosa or corneal blindness. He was right; the operation was an improvement in that regard, but it still fell well short of ideal. Disturbing postoperative facial numbness was still a problem, and so surgeons continued their quest for the Golden Grail of TN surgery—an operation that would cure the pain without permanently damaging the trigeminal nerve—well into the latter half of the twentieth century.

In the 1950s surgeons began acting on Dandy's theory of vascular nerve compression and devised methods for moving the offending arteries away from the trigeminal nerve at the point where it entered the brain. At first, arteries were simply repositioned; later, in the 1960s, surgeons began wrapping the nerve with gelatin, muscle, or woven plastic sponges to prevent the repositioned arteries from finding their way back against the damaged nerve. The results were excellent, producing pain relief lasting five to ten years in the majority of patients and, best of all, with little numbness and scant risk of anesthesia dolorosa.

The operation came to be known as microvascular decompression (the delicate mobilization of arteries requires an operating microscope). Although Dandy discovered the cause of TN and other surgeons (notably the late James Gardner of Cleveland Clinic) perfected the technique of moving the blood vessels away from the nerve, microvascular decompression became identified with my old mentor, Peter Jannetta. Jannetta, due largely to his avuncular charisma and prodigious operative skill, almost single-handedly changed microvascular decompression from an obscure procedure into a mainstream sensation. He traveled the world doing and teaching the procedure and became a fixture at international meetings. By the early 1970s the "Jannetta procedure," as it came to be known, was the operation of choice for TN. Although newer, less-invasive methods for treating the pain have since been developed, the procedure remains a viable therapy to the present day.

❧

We operated on Mildred many years ago, and I no longer remember who actually did her surgery, Jannetta or one of his many assistants. But I was there.

She was near death's door when I first met her. She was emaciated, her blue eyes dull and sunken. She looked like a cancer patient without the cancer; her lips were pursed and she drew her breaths slowly and with exquisite care. Over the years she had learned just how fast the air could flow past her gums before the pains came. Sometimes, desperate for oxygen, she would suck in a large breath and then yelp, bringing her hand quickly to her face but stopping it just short of contact, never allowing the hand to touch her cheek. She was like a martial arts master I once knew who could throw a vicious punch at me but stop an inch short of actually striking my face. Several years of practice had given Mildred the same degree of arm control.

Years later I found out firsthand what Mildred must have been going through. As I was seeing patients one Friday afternoon, I foolishly paused to chew a caramel candy and promptly pulled a large filling out of one of my rear molars. With a large portion of the tooth's nerve now exposed, I found that I could barely breathe without excruciating stabs of jaw pain. I tried to rinse some of the candy away with lukewarm water and nearly passed out. Unable to speak and barely able to swallow, I canceled my patients and headed straight to a dentist's office. My life as a TN patient lasted less than two hours; Mildred's had lasted for three years.

As I discussed with her the formidable risks involved with manipulating the arteries of her brain, she just nodded, eyes closed. Melodramatic as it may sound, when I'm alone with a chronic pain patient, it feels as though three entities are in that room: the patient, the pain, and me. So palpable is the pain, even to an outsider, that it becomes another living creature to deal with, not a disease to be treated but a conscious demon to be exorcised. Mildred quickly signed the consent form and brusquely motioned for me to leave so that she could be alone with her pain, that constant and unwanted companion.

At surgery we found Mildred's right trigeminal nerve bent awkwardly over a cerebellar artery. The nerve, splayed over the thick calcified vessel, had been thinned to less than half of its normal diameter by years of arterial pounding. We moved the vessel away and a shoved a small piece of plastic sponge between it and the nerve. Mildred awakened free of face pain and remained that way until I last saw her, about a year after her surgery. She now talked freely, years of sentences rolling out in great pent-up waves. She now spoke of grandchildren whom she hadn't been able to talk to or kiss for so long...and the tears came again. She couldn't say whether they were tears of joy or tears of mourning—mourning for the long and irretrievable period that TN had carved from her life.

I haven't seen her since, but most patients stay pain free, or nearly so, for a long time. And I'm sure she would have sought us out had her pain returned. I was happy that Mildred ended up with "the face she deserved," a face free of pain. With the help of surgery, Mildred tossed aside the phantom's mask of torment that made her an exile from life and was able to at last escape the opera house of her pain.

~

Unfortunately, the story of TN doesn't always have a happy ending, and the dramatic saga of microvascular decompression turns out to have an unexpected plot twist. Yes, *most* patients stay pain free after the Jannetta procedure, but not *all.* Up to 40 percent of TN patients experience a recurrence of pain within the first decade following microvascular decompression of their trigeminal nerves. Luckily, the pain is rarely as frequent or as severe as it was prior to surgery, and many patients will respond to a second or even a third decompression operation. Of course, a decade of relief may be all that some patients require given the advanced age of many TN sufferers.

But the fact that *any* patients recur is troubling and raises serious doubts about the validity of Dandy's vascular compression theory—or at least about the rationale for microvascular decompression. If arterial compression of the nerve is the sole cause of TN, removing the arterial compression should produce a lasting cure, but it doesn't. If the operation is repeated, a few patients will be found to have new arterial compression of their nerve, but most do not. Why does the pain recur? We still don't know for sure. The trigeminal nerve may be permanently damaged by the original arterial compression, such that surgery to remove the artery may not cure everyone. Mildred's nerve had been reduced to half of its normal size and would probably never be "normal" again, even if it never bothered her. If a pickup truck runs over my foot, the foot may hurt long after the offending tire rolls away.

But if permanent nerve injury is to blame for the operation's delayed failures, why do the vast majority of patients get well immediately and stay well for years, only to relapse a decade or more later? Patients with irreparable nerve damage should never improve at all, with or without surgery. In the pickup truck analogy, if my foot is wrecked by being run over, I should know it right away. I shouldn't walk normally after the tire comes off my foot only to begin limping years later.

There is another troubling paradox in the Dandy theory: If the painful paroxysms of TN are the result of arterial injury to the nerve, why do patients like Mildred wake up from surgery free of pain? The nerve will need weeks, maybe many months, to repair itself, yet pain relief occurs instantaneously after nerve decompression. How does this happen?

But should we question our success? After all, the Jannetta procedure produces immediate pain relief in over nine out of ten patients and long-term relief in two out of three. The answer is yes, we can question this success. Although highly effective, the operation comes with a hefty price tag in the form of serious complications. Manipulation of critical brain arteries buried within a nest of sensitive cranial nerves carries with it a significant risk of crippling postoperative strokes, deafness, facial paralysis, coma, and death. These are not theoretical risks; they have all happened. The need for hours of brain surgery under general anesthesia also limits the use of microvascular decompression to relatively healthy patients. Very elderly or infirm TN sufferers may not be eligible for decompression at all.

Early hopes that Jannetta's vaunted operation represented the long-awaited cure for TN soon waned. The high risks of the Jannetta procedure and a growing appreciation of its disappointing long-term recurrence rate spurred surgeons to resume their search for a better TN operation, one that didn't require opening the head or playing with the brain. In the 1980s two promising new candidates emerged: glycerol injection and balloon microcompression. Both are throwbacks to the earlier needle procedures.

Glycerol is a mild alcohol that selectively destroys those nerve fibers lacking myelin (pain fibers) while preserving myelin-coated fibers (touch fibers). When injected into the trigeminal nerve through the cheek, glycerol kills the trigeminal pain fibers but leaves touch fibers intact, yielding good pain relief and only minimal numbness. This is a clear example of how the differential anatomy of pain and fine touch can be exploited therapeutically. In the balloon microcompression technique, a tiny uninflated balloon is threaded through a thick needle into the nerve. Once in proper position, the balloon is inflated for several minutes, gently compressing the nerve. Why this modest mechanical crushing action should relieve TN pain remains unclear, but it works. Once again, good pain relief without significant numbness can be achieved. In fact, both glycerol and balloon microcompression produce results almost (but not quite) comparable to the more dangerous Jannetta technique. Glycerol injection can be done under fairly painless local anesthesia, while balloon microcompression requires anesthetizing the patient. However, both are brief and relatively risk free.

The similar results obtained with microvascular decompression, glycerol injection, and balloon microcompression suggest that all three procedures produce pain relief through a common mechanism: nerve damage. Although nerve damage isn't the rationale for the Jannetta procedure, the operation, even in skilled hands, will indeed injure the trigeminal nerve. Elegant as microvascular decompression sounds in theory, in practice there is nothing particularly gentle about pulling an adherent blood vessel away from the nerve, then exposing the nerve to the drying action of air, heating it with an electrocautery, and finally rubbing it with a plastic sponge. The instant pain relief observed after microvascular decompression most likely results from mild operative nerve injury and not from the decompression itself. (The efficacy of the more recently developed balloon microcompression technique shows how little trauma is needed to stop TN for years at a time.) Since no ablative procedure works forever, microvascular decompression, like other nerve injuries, will only produce temporary relief.

Thus, we haven't escaped Dandy's paradigm at all but have instead returned full circle to the nineteenth-century maxim: To treat TN surgically, we must damage the nerve, at least a tiny bit. But we've become more selective about how we do this. By using more gentle techniques, we can relieve pain and still avoid the devastating problems of total nerve destruction. Coagulating or cutting the entire nerve is like dropping an atom bomb on a country just to get rid of a few miscreants. Procedures like microvascular decompression, glycerol injection, and balloon microcompression are smart bombs, targeting just the pain pathways while leaving the more vital touch pathways unharmed.

Dandy's theory is still likely to be the correct one; vascular compression and the resultant nerve injury probably do cause most TN. But the operation spawned by his theory—microvascular decompression—although quite useful, may not work in the way its inventors thought it would. Although it removes the cause of TN, microvascular decompression doesn't cure the illness at all, but only ameliorates it by inflicting a mild trauma to the nerve. The belief that we could undo years of nerve damage in a surgical instant was, in retrospect, overly optimistic.

Presently, many surgeons still prefer microvascular decompression in patients who fail drug therapy, because it gives the best results, irrespective of how it works. Other surgeons prefer to begin with glycerol injection or balloon microcompression, holding the riskier Jannetta operation in reserve and using it only if the smaller procedures fail. I favor the latter course. Although I make my living doing brain surgery, I have learned that it's best not to disturb the magnificent machine between our ears unless absolutely necessary.

There is one additional option, one that involves no surgery: stereotactic radiation of the nerve. Currently being investigated by an old colleague of mine, Doug Kondziolka of the University of Pittsburgh, stereotactic radiosurgery uses computer-guided cobalt radiation to create precise injuries within the head and brain. The device that accomplishes this is called a gamma knife because it uses gamma rays with surgical accuracy. Devised in the 1950s by the late Swedish neurosurgeon Lars Leksell, the gamma knife is now commonly used to destroy small tumors and vascular malformations, even though Leksell originally hoped to treat TN. Kondziolka is now, four decades later, trying to accomplish this. So far, radiation-induced trigeminal damage looks promising, but the results are still too preliminary to draw any conclusions about a more widespread role for the gamma knife in TN management.

The final answer to neuropathic craniofacial pain syndromes will not likely come from surgeons but from molecular biologists. Curing these illnesses will require some way of restoring the integrity of damaged nerves at the microscopic level. As the old Sanskrit proverb states, the fox has many good tricks but the hedgehog has one great trick. The reason we have many good methods of treating TN—carbamazine, microvascular compression, gamma knife, glycerol injection, balloon microcompression—is that we lack one great method. We once believed that Jannetta would be our hedgehog and teach us that method, but that now seems unlikely. Until a new "great trick" arises, we must rely on our good ones—the flawed drugs and invasive operations that, although far from perfect, can still make the Mildreds of the world smile painlessly once more.

4 THE HUMAN AFFLICTION

I have everything I had twenty years ago—except now, it's all lower.

—Gypsy Rose Lee

Anne first entered my exam room with the aid of a beach towel slung beneath her right knee. Using the towel like a puppeteer's string, she raised and lowered her leg manually as she walked; the limb was too painful and wobbly to function unassisted. Anne, a realtor in her late forties, laughed heartily when I told her that she looked like a large marionette. "Yes," she replied, "a regular Howdy Doody."

Anne told me that she was working in her garden the previous week when her problems first began. Although she had experienced some mild back pain on and off for a few weeks, she felt something truly unusual as she stooped to hoist a small bag of black topsoil. As she straightened up, she heard a sickening pop in her lower back and within minutes her thigh and shin began buzzing—a weird electrical sensation that felt like a toy train transformer had been hooked to her skin. Later that day the buzz turned into mild pain radiating from the hip and down the leg. She also felt a faint weakness in the thigh as she climbed the stairs to her bedroom that night. The following morning she could barely move. The small ember of discomfort she had felt the evening before now billowed into a flame engulfing much of her leg. She was soon unable to walk without the aid of her towel.

I knew at first glance what was wrong with Anne. Her curious gait belied the mundane nature of her illness. She suffered from that uniquely human affliction known as the herniated lumbar spinal disc (aka the "ruptured" or "slipped" disc). Although her story suggested that her illness was barely one week old, I knew that Anne's disc problem, like almost all disc problems, had really started decades earlier. As we will see, the seeds of disc rupture are sewn in our twenties or, in some cases, even earlier.

The colloquial term for leg pain arising from a ruptured lumbar disc is sciatica, a word coined by Shakespeare in his play *Timon of Athens.* ("Thou couldst, sciatica, cripple our senators as lamely as their manners.") Shakespeare clearly subscribed to the notion that sciatica arose from the thick sciatic nerve (from the Greek *ischiadikos,* for "hip"). The nerve lies buried in the buttock and posterior thigh, and since pain felt by victims follows the precise course of the nerve, this misconception made good sense. The Bard was not alone in that belief. Amazingly, medical science didn't discover the real cause of sciatica—inflamed nerves in the lumbar spine, not in the leg—until the middle part of this century, almost three hundred years after Shakespeare first named the condition.

During her initial office visit, I prescribed for Anne a regimen of steroids, analgesics, and physical therapy lasting for several weeks. Her leg weakness was too mild to consider back surgery to correct the disc rupture right away. I also ordered a magnetic resonance scan of her lumbar spine, which neatly displayed the source of her problem. As I expected, a tiny fragment from inside one of the discs in her lower lumbar spine had broken free and was now wedged against her fourth lumbar nerve root, a spaghetti-sized cable destined for her thigh and shin areas. The piece of dislocated disc was small, barely larger than a pencil eraser, but sat squarely and stubbornly on the irritated nerve root. Only time would tell if Anne's body could digest this offending fragment by itself; otherwise, I would be called upon to extract it in the operating room.

The human spine stands bolt upright for two-thirds of its existence; as such, the soft discs situated between adjacent vertebrae must endure the full brunt of our upper body weight as we sit, stand, or walk. The constant compressive forces exerted on the discs by our erect posture puts them at greater risk of rupture compared to the discs of quadriped animals. To add insult to injury, we top off this erect human spine with an absurdly heavy head, which sits perched on the tiny neck bones like a bowling ball atop a broomstick. It amazes me that our spines hold up as well as they do.

Spinal disc disorders are approaching epidemic numbers in industrialized nations; about one in every four adults will know the pain of sciatica during their lifetimes. This may have something to do with our growing tendency toward obesity and our increasingly sedentary lifestyle. Excessive body weight can stress weakened discs to the breaking point. Moreover, by allowing our back and abdominal muscles to grow slack, we also force the discs to carry more than their fair share of the load.

A distinction must be made here between low back pain of muscular origin and sciatica of disc origin. Almost three-quarters of the population suffer from recurring episodes of moderate to severe low back pain, but these episodes most often arise in fatigued muscles or strained ligaments and have nothing to do with the bones or discs of the spinal column itself. Paradoxically, back pain may not be prominent in true sciatica, even though the spine is the epicenter of the problem. Anne, for example, had only minor back discomfort throughout the course of her illness.

✦

A typical spinal disc consists of a moist core (the nucleus pulposus) encased by a shell of coarse fibrous tissue (the annulus). Because they have semiliquid centers and tough, flexible hides, discs resemble flattened golf balls; this compressible design allows them to serve as shock absorbers, smoothing the bumpy ride between the vertebrae. When healthy, a disc can withstand hundreds of pounds of force without breaking apart, just as a new golf ball can withstand massive blows from metal clubs without exploding.

Discs are built from cartilage, ligament, and elastic fibers—biological building blocks collectively known as connective tissues because they connect us, or hold us together. Connective tissues are the duct tape and mortar of the human body and are remarkably strong; ounce for ounce as strong as the toughest plastics.

But connective tissues don't stay strong forever. Shortly after puberty, they begin a slow, age-dependent deterioration that results in progressive loss of their moisture, strength, and elasticity. In short, our structural tissues grow drier, weaker, and more brittle with age. Among the first structures to manifest this aging are the discs, which can start to weaken in our late teens or early twenties.

Most patients are astounded to learn that disc disease can occur in any adult, even at a young age; many people believe that only the senior population or those engaged in heavy labor have trouble with their discs. To help my patients understand the ubiquitous nature of disc deterioration, I point out that the lenses in their eyes are anatomically similar to the discs in their spines. The lens, like the disc, is an elastic sac of connective tissue.

Between the ages of thirty and sixty, we develop a progressive inability to focus on nearby objects, a condition known as presbyopia. It's the reason we all need reading glasses eventually. It comes to some people sooner, others later, but everyone who lives long enough gets it. Presbyopia is caused by the same deterioration of our connective tissues that is responsible for bad discs.

The aging of our connective tissues is apparent in other parts of the body, too. As Gypsy Rose Lee wryly observed, those parts of our external anatomy that require strong connective tissues to support them—such as our facial skin, breasts, abdomen, and buttocks—begin to sag noticeably in the fourth and fifth decades. Although the sagging of these structures hurts us cosmetically, the concomitant sagging of our internal support systems can predispose us to serious pain, as Anne abruptly discovered.

The sagging of an aging disc is more properly known as disc degeneration. As the degenerating discs dry out and lose their youthful elastic tone, they tend to bulge out at the sides like underinflated tires (the so-called bulging disc phenomenon). The stretching of the disc's outer wall (annulus) caused by this bulging can cause occasional low-level back discomfort and, more importantly, weakens the annulus, predisposing it to ripping open and spilling out the disc's inner core.

Not all of our discs degenerate at the same pace. The typical spine has twenty-four discs but only two in the lumbar spine and three in the neck show major signs of degeneration in the average lifetime. These five discs account for over 90 percent of all clinical disc problems—including Anne's—largely because they reside in the most mobile areas of our spines.

Discs suffer their greatest strain during spinal flexion. For example, when we bend forward at the waist, the vertebrae in our lower lumbar spine act like the jaws of a vice, compressing the intervening discs. Pressure-measuring devices inserted into the spines of normal volunteers confirm the extraordinary strain placed on the lumbar discs during the simple act of leaning over a sink to wash dishes (although I've always wondered why anyone would "volunteer" to have measuring devices inserted into their spines). These studies also have a deeper lesson: Avoid washing dishes at every opportunity.

Flexion, or bending, only takes place in the lower neck and lower lumbar area. The rib cage prevents bending of the chest region (the thoracic spine). Consequently, thoracic discs take so little stress that they rarely rupture.

We know that repeated mechanical stress accelerates the degenerative process. That's why many people have prosthetic knee and hip joints but few will ever need prosthetic elbow or wrist joints. Although all joints are prone to deterioration, weight-bearing joints like the hips and knees age faster than non-weight-bearing joints like elbows and wrists. The same is true in the spine. Those parts of the spine that take the most mechanical pounding, namely the lower lumbar spine and the lower neck, wear out faster. Thus, spinal disc disease is the result of two simultaneous processes: a genetically programmed aging of the disc's constituent connective tissues and cumulative wear and tear caused by repetitive spinal flexion.

➤

Disc degeneration is not the same thing as disc herniation. A disc herniates when the disc's weakened annulus splits open and allows some of its gelatinous inner core, the nucleus pulposus, to ooze out like toothpaste squirting through a rent in the metal tube. In the lingo of spine experts, this event is called an HNP— herniated nucleus pulposus. The herniated material, which at surgery resembles lump crabmeat, can wind up pressing on nearby spinal nerves and creating terrible pain radiating in the distribution of those nerves: into the legs in the case of herniated lumbar discs or into the arms in the case of herniated discs in the neck.

Healthy discs are much too strong to rupture unless subjected to extreme forces, and years of disc degeneration almost always precede clinical sciatica. The forces needed to rupture a young disc approach those capable of snapping the spine itself in two. For example, I once cared for a young pilot who ruptured a normal thoracic disc, ejecting from his fighter plane after his engine failed. Pulling ten g's can do that, but lifting a small bag of dirt can't. In order for Anne's disc to break apart after lifting a few pounds of soil, the annulus had to be compromised by years of disc deterioration and wear. Thus, a disc herniation is like a heart attack, the final catastrophic event in a degenerative process years in the making.

The fact that her disc disease didn't start on the day she lifted her bag of soil may not seem important at first glance. Consider, however, that an entire multibillion-dollar liability industry has sprung up around spinal disc disease in the United States alone. If Anne had been lifting a FOR SALE sign at one of the houses she was selling when her disc ruptured, she could have sued her employer for medical bills and lost wages and would have almost certainly won. She might even be able to claim that her back condition would never allow her to work again and thus retire on the company's payroll. From a medical point of view, this is silly. Her back disease did not stem from any one incident; the disc was degenerating and prone to rupture at the appropriate provocation. It was a worn tire ready to blow. But the current civil liability system looks at disc disease as being "caused" by isolated lifting or falling injuries when, in truth, it is a ubiquitous consequence of aging. Heavy lifting doesn't cause disc disease any more than shoveling snow causes heart disease. These activities merely trigger a rapid decompensation of an already diseased organ.

Disc degeneration in the absence of frank herniation can cause occasional backaches and morning stiffness, but this discomfort is rarely long lasting or incapacitating. Frequently, disc degeneration alone produces no symptoms at all. A recent study of adults with no history of back problems found that almost half of them had at least one markedly degenerating lumbar disc on magnetic resonance scanning. Thus, the most significant problem associated with degenerating discs is their heightened risk of rupture.

When rupture does occur, it's almost always associated with severe and acute pain, except in odd cases where the herniated disc fragment ends up in some harmless place, such as in the adjoining vertebral bone or the abdomen. Thanks to an unfortunate design flaw, herniated disc debris typically goes backward into the path of exiting spinal nerves. In the normal spine, these sensitive nerves lie barely a quarter of an inch from the adjoining discs. The close proximity of the fragile spinal discs to the spinal nerves makes sciatica the epidemic problem that it is. If the discs and nerves weren't so closely approximated, our discs could herniate on a daily basis and we wouldn't care.

How did this unfortunate anatomy evolve? Why were the spine's shock absorbers, so prone to wearing out and breaking apart, placed right up against our nerves? The juxtaposition is so intimate that even the most minuscule extrusion of disc material has the capacity to cause crippling nerve pain. Not that I'm complaining, of course. As a disc surgeon for most of my life, this bizarre spinal architecture has kept food on my family's table for many years.

Why do we have the disease-prone spines that we do? First, we must remember that evolution has no mercy and doesn't care if we have pain so long as that pain doesn't permanently cripple us or kill us before we've had the opportunity to reproduce. Ruptured discs are painful but not lethal, and they tend to run their course in a few weeks. Moreover, bad discs are more of a problem for those of us beyond our peak childbearing years.

We must also remember that the basic layout of the spine evolved a hundred million years ago for animals maintaining a largely horizontal posture. It's no exaggeration to say that evolving humans simply took a horizontally designed backbone and jacked it upright with little modification. Go to a local museum and observe the backbone of a stegosaurus—it's basically the same as ours. However, in the case of the stegosaurus (or the cow, for that matter), the enormous weight of the animal was directed *perpendicular* to the axis of the spine, the body weight hanging down from the backbone like wet laundry from a clothesline, putting little pressure on the discs. In the human design, our body weight is directed parallel to our spinal axis, a radical change. Using a horizontal spinal architecture for vertical walking is like using a screwdriver to drive nails: the nails may get driven, but a lot of screwdrivers will be shattered in the process. The price we pay for our new posture? Lots of shattered discs.

Since we've only been using our newly upright spines for a few hundred thousand years—a mere blink of a Darwinian eye—there has been no time for natural selection to work out all of the kinks inherent in such a radical reorientation of the spine. Thus, I see sciatica as the curse of early hominids like us. Fortunately, evolution didn't abandon us entirely. Our erect posture damages our spines but also frees our hands, giving us one way to compensate for our rupturing discs: we can now become surgeons and remove them.

➤

Anne left my office dragging her recalcitrant leg behind her and started physical therapy several days later. The steroid pills would help reduce the inflammation in her ailing lumbar nerve and the narcotic pain medications would help her cope with the pain in the short term.

Physicians tend to prescribe physical therapy as the initial treatment of herniated discs. Left to their own devices, patients more often seek out chiropractors. I have found that the distinction between conventional physical therapy and chiropractic has blurred over the years, as physical therapists start to employ chiropractic spinal manipulations and chiropractors begin using

some of the tools of the therapists. Both disciplines are fair at relieving back pain, but neither achieves consistent success when
attempting to treat the sciatica that emanates from compressed
spinal nerves.

In reality, time is the best medicine for most disc herniations.
Over two-thirds of patients will feel their pain diminish to tolerable levels (or vanish totally) within a month of their acute herniations; even in the absence of any therapy, three-quarters
improve within three months. Most will never require surgical
removal of the offending disc fragment. The ancient Greek
physician Hippocrates once said that medicine is the art of en-
tertaining people until they heal themselves, and that's largely
what medications, physical therapy, chiropractic, and steroids do
for acute disc patients—entertain but do not cure. There is no
evidence that these therapies, or any therapy short of surgery, re-
store the disc's integrity or in any way treat the problem in a
structural sense. The goal of treatment is to keep the victim
comfortable until his or her pain abates on its own. If the pain
doesn't ease in a reasonable amount of time or if the affected
nerve shows signs of injury in the form of major limb weakness,
numbness, or bladder dysfunction, then surgery to decompress
the nerve and remove the fragmented disc must be considered.

Why does the pain go away? A smashed nerve should be a
smashed nerve forever, but the body does find ways to heal itself,
a good thing considering that we've been rupturing discs for
thousands of years but only operating on them recently. In some
cases the extruded piece of disc material is absorbed and the
nerve becomes slowly decompressed. In effect, the body performs
spinal surgery upon itself (and without preapproval from an
HMO, I might add).

In other cases the disc remains ruptured perpetually, yet the nerve learns to ignore the permanent distortion created by the recalcitrant disc. No one has a clue how this miracle happens, but it does. Finally, a badly pinched nerve may simply die off, leaving the patient with numbness but happily free of pain. The last scenario is akin to a root canal. During a root canal, the dentist avulses a suffering dental nerve to alleviate tooth pain. In like fashion, some discs destroy a spinal nerve altogether, also relieving the pain.

Unfortunately Anne's physical therapy only made her worse, and within a week of her first visit she was calling and begging me to do something, anything. The pain had become so severe that it actually had made her vomit on two occasions. Despite the incessant warnings of her friends that back surgery would only "ruin her" forever, Anne reached the point that amputation of the leg would have been welcome to halt the leg pain. I admitted her to the hospital and planned to do her surgery the following morning.

Surgery for herniated discs is a simpleminded affair. Although most operations are fairly simpleminded, disc removal, or discectomy, is particularly simpleminded: a piece of disc is crushing a nerve, so the surgeon must remove that piece. Simple. The standard disc operation (also known as the dreaded "back operation") involves opening the skin and muscles overlying the spine with a knife, drilling a window in the thin plate of bone protecting the spinal nerves, and removing the offending fragments of herniated disc with long forceps. The bone covering the nerves is called the lamina, Latin for "layer" (think of laminated wood), and its removal is called a laminectomy. The words *laminectomy* and *discectomy* can be used interchangeably, even though the discectomy is the heart and soul of the procedure. The operation is also called an "open" discectomy because it requires opening the spine and removing the disc under direct vision.

The discectomy was invented by Drs. Mixter and Barr about fifty years ago and has evolved into one of the most frequently performed operations in developed nations. In their early incarnations, open discectomies required enormous incisions, massive bone removal, and prolonged recuperative times—up to six months. In its present form, used since the early 1970s, the microdiscectomy, as it's now known, requires a skin incision less than two inches in length, the removal of a dime-sized piece of bone, and a recovery period of a month or less. An experienced surgeon can judge in which decade a patient underwent back surgery by the length of the scar. Incisions dating back to the 1950s can be a foot or more in length.

Recently a slew of even smaller procedures has been developed to eliminate the need for open surgery and general anesthesia altogether. For example, in the 1980s the enzyme chymopapain was injected into diseased discs to shrink them. Derived from the papaya plant, chymopapain digests disc cartilage, and its proponents argued that this would eliminate open disc surgery forever. Unfortunately for them (and for some of their patients), chymopapain, a key ingredient in many meat tenderizers, also dissolved other tissues, including muscles and nerves, and the procedure has fallen out of favor because of its unsatisfactory outcomes.

Also in the 1980s, percutaneous discectomy appeared. Percutaneous surgeons insert a long, thin metal tube under X-ray guidance into the affected disc and remove disc substance, using a twirling mechanical blade or a laser beam. Although it sounds high-tech, the percutaneous disc device operates on the same principle as a plumber's snake. It's basically a chewing device fixed to the end of a long stick. As I said, this is simpleminded stuff.

My mother says that I was born forty years old, and this conservative streak shows in my clinical practice. If I'm going to be waving sharp instruments around spinal nerves, I prefer to see what I'm doing. For that reason, I have rejected the minimal operations and offer prospective surgical patients only open discectomy. Although it requires a longer hospital stay and a more protracted recovery period, the open discectomy yields the best long-term pain relief. In the final analysis, that's what people really want, anyway. What good is a smaller incision or shorter hospital stay if you're still in pain?

⇌

Anne's surgery went smoothly. I found her fourth lumbar nerve stretched tautly over a lump of wayward disc material. I pushed the swollen nerve gently away from the disc fragment and pulled the piece of glistening cartilage out of the spine. I then tossed the source of her pain into a silver basin to be whisked away forever. An instant cure. I could almost hear the nerve sighing in relief. I probed about a bit more and located the rip in her disc's annulus that gave rise to the herniation in the first place. It was large, about the diameter of a ballpoint pen. There's no easy way to repair these large holes, so surgeons routinely enter the center of the disc and try to scrape away what's left of the disc's interior in order to prevent more nucleous pulposus from extruding later on.

During the typical disc rupture, less than 10 percent of the nucleous pulposus oozes out. At surgery the surgeon can, at best, remove another 50 percent. That leaves a little less than half of the nucleous to cause more problems in the future. It's just too dangerous to clean out the entire disc, not because the spine will fall apart (it won't), but because the disc is surrounded by large arteries and veins and an aggressive disc removal can cause the patient to bleed to death. Thus, despite our most strenuous efforts, patients have about a one in six chance of herniating the same disc through the same annular hole at some point in the future, even after adequate surgical therapy. I've had patients reherniate their discs before they've even left the recovery room from the first operations. That's why everyone knows old Uncle Joe or some guy down the street who needed three back operations. Of course, everyone blames the surgeon, which is wrong. The nature of the disease is to recur, and no safe operation can prevent this.

Can anything prevent disc deterioration? My patients often ask what lifestyle adjustments they can make to delay the onset of a new disc problem or prevent the recurrence of a prior one. There are three adjustments they can make, but none of them is easy.

First and foremost: Lose weight. If a car's shock absorbers are bad, don't use it to haul pianos. Carrying two hundred pounds on a skeleton meant to carry one hundred and fifty will accelerate disc degeneration.

Second, get into excellent physical shape and, in particular, strengthen the abdominal muscles. To understand how a strong abdomen takes stress off the discs, consider an old grade school science experiment: Start with a few hundred sheets of ordinary typing paper. Roll and tape them into tubes, then tape all of the tubes together into a honeycomb pattern and place a piece of plywood on top of the honeycomb. Four or five people can now stand on the plywood platform, effectively standing on the rolled edges of flimsy paper sheets without the paper collapsing. This experiment demonstrates how even a weak material can become very strong when rolled into tubes. That's why a long wrapping paper tube is so much stiffer than the cardboard from which it's made.

A muscular torso is like the cardboard tube: strong and rigid, and capable of supporting the body even without a spine (this is no exaggeration—cadavers of muscular men will sit upright even after the spine has been removed). A torso devoid of tone, on the other hand, must depend solely upon the rigid structures of the spine for its support.

The third and final lifestyle adjustment that can aid an aching spine is the cessation of smoking. Cigarette smoking accelerates the aging of all of our connective tissues. Anyone who doubts this need only compare the faces of adult smokers to those of non-smokers. Heavy smokers show relatively greater loss of skin elasticity and increased wrinkling. In short, they look older than nonsmokers of equal chronological age. The same accelerated aging affects the discs of smokers as well. This isn't speculative; studies confirm that smokers have more problems with disc disease and respond less well to disc surgery.

Lose weight, exercise, and don't smoke. That's the best we can do. The rest is genetics. And, of course, luck.

***

Anne woke up with her pain about "80 percent" relieved, to use her own estimate. Very few people are completely free of all leg pain in the first days and weeks after successful disc surgery. As anyone who has had a crown put on a tooth can verify, irritated nerves don't settle down overnight. Anne did leave the hospital sans towel, which was a major victory. Her pain didn't leave entirely until about five or six weeks after surgery, and it was three months before she could walk up stairs normally again. She's now recovered and back to gardening and selling houses. I haven't heard from her in years and that's fine with me. With disc patients, no news is good news.

Despite the fact that it can work near miracles in terms of rapid pain relief, discectomy remains a much-maligned operation. Two friends who tried dissuading Anne from going ahead with surgery—the ones who claimed she would be ruined by it—visited her the afternoon following her operation and were amazed at how well she was doing. I asked if either of them had ever had sciatica and both sheepishly replied no. How sad, I thought. A painless person discouraging a suffering friend from surgery is like a well-fed person discouraging a starving man from eating out of Dumpsters. What seems nasty to one person may be another's salvation.

Critics of discectomy point to the wide geographic variability in discectomy rates, arguing that the surgery is driven by the greed of surgeons more than by the pain of their patients. In some parts of California and Florida, for example, eight out of every one thousand adults will eventually undergo back surgery. In some parts of the Midwest, the surgery rate drops to a mere one or two per thousand. Do Californians and Floridians rupture their discs eight times more frequently than midwesterners or, as the critics contend, is there something more sinister going on here?

Something is going on all right, but it's hardly sinister.

Discectomy is a "quality of life" operation, meaning that it's done to enhance life, not prolong it. In this regard, discectomy is like a face-lift. Face-lifts are invasive, risky operations done for one purpose, namely to allow the people to feel better about themselves. No one needs a face-lift in a medical sense. Likewise, many people *want* discectomies, as Anne did, but few *need* them.

Rarely do victims of disc herniations suffer the degree of pain Anne felt and so most patients aren't forced into having surgery. Moreover, most patients get better on their own eventually, provided they sit around long enough eating pain pills. But how much pain is too much? And how much waiting before bailing out and choosing surgery is enough? These are subjective matters that will vary in different patient populations. Some people will ask for surgery sooner than others; some people can tolerate pain better than others. I doubt that I would have earned much of a living doing pain surgery in ancient Sparta, but in a community composed largely of type A urban professionals who believe that every shred of their pain should have been gone yesterday, I stay busy.

Granted, I speak from a highly biased perspective, but of all pain-relieving modalities ever used in the history of medicine— including narcotics, cordotomy, acupuncture, snake oil, whatever—simple open discectomy provides the greatest pain relief for the least long-term risk. I still relish the look on a patient's face when he or she awakens from anesthesia free of misery.

That's what I live for professionally. I consider it an honor to keep us silly, bulbous-headed hominids walking upright, as unnatural as that may be.

5   A WOMAN'S WAR

While she was berrying
She bore that child...
And sprang forward, screaming
To terrify that child

—from an Alaskan Indian birth poem

"Breathe. Breathe. Breathe."

I repeated this mantra again and again as my wife fought to maintain her composure. Writhing in the throes of her increasingly ferocious uterine contractions, she labored with our first daughter as I watched, powerless to assist her. As chief neurosurgical resident of a large urban medical center, I could barely find a few idle hours in a day to sleep let alone participate in weekly Lamaze classes. One of our friends who had training as a Lamaze instructor gave us a crash course in natural childbirth techniques a few days earlier, but that brief exposure proved of little use in the heat of the moment. My wife wanted to deliver without anesthesia, the so-called "natural" way. Unfortunately, neither of us knew what we were doing and her pain soon spiraled out of control.

I sat slouched in an unpadded metal chair. That chair was a torture device; I was convinced that the OB nurse forced me to sit in it so that I, too, could suffer. My wife squirmed in her sweaty bed as I squirmed in that sweaty chair, two anxious people locked in a slow, joyless dance. I longed for the old days, when dads-to-be smoked and paced in the waiting room far removed from the drama of the birthing suite.

"Breathe!" I yelled again, but I didn't understand what these exhortations were supposed to accomplish. Telling a woman on the verge of passing out from hyperventilation to breathe is like leaning over the *Titanic's* tilting deck rail and screaming, "Drown!" to those bobbing in the sea. What else can they do?

She calmed down as each contraction ended, but her anticipation of pain magnified with each successive spasm of her impatient womb. Hours passed and she grew dreadfully weary, her face moist and gray like the mask of someone approaching death. I had seen the same look many times before, the expression of a body pushed to its physiologic limit, and this appearance frightened me. The painless intervals grew shorter and the contractions lengthened, the normal progression of advancing labor. She wanted desperately to hang on and complete the "natural" process of birthing, but she finally realized that this pain could not continue. About seven hours into her labor, an anesthesiologist arrived at our request and inserted an epidural catheter into her back, a thin tube placed near the nerves of the lumbar spine. An infusion of spinal narcotic immediately deadened the pelvic area and uterus. Without the violent effects of pain to drive it forward, her labor slowed down slightly, but things eventually came to fruition with the birth of a screaming infant girl.

Because epidural anesthesia produces no sedation, my wife was still able to cooperate fully with the delivery. She didn't see the actual birth (my large head blocked her view of the mirror, a fact I'm not permitted to forget even ten years later), but she managed to hold her new child immediately. Both mother and child were bright and alert. In my wife's case, abandoning natural birth in favor of an epidural block did nothing to harm the birthing experience. In fact, the spinal narcotics enhanced it; by sparing my wife hours of agony, the epidural catheter allowed her to meet her new daughter in a rested and refreshed state. Emily proved to be a normal, healthy child and my wife recovered quickly and without problems. What more could anyone ask of childbirth?

Nevertheless, my wife harbored twinges of doubt concerning her performance, as if her first labor, although successful in outcome, was marred by some measure of personal failure because it was not natural in the strictest sense of the word. I, too, felt guilty about the epidural block. I considered my wife's plea for anesthesia to be my fault, not hers. After all, I hadn't made time in my schedule to learn how to coach a natural childbirth correctly, even though she had asked me to do so on numerous occasions. I wasn't prepared to do my part to assist her, to talk her through the ordeal without resorting to drugs and needles.

Looking back on that event of years ago, I'm somewhat mystified over this guilt. What's so bad about a comfortable labor and delivery, even one that required medical technology? In the historical scheme of things, I did nothing wrong. Prior to this century, childbirth was rarely a team sport. In those instances when expectant mothers needed the assistance of others, they sought out experienced women, not nervous and useless fathers.

Men view childbirth only as a process that produces their children. To women, of course, it's more—much more. Childbirth is a profound ritual teeming with spiritual and biological significance. Pain appears to play an indispensable role in that ritual. In the words of poet Helen Chasin:

Screwed on this centripetal ache, I fix on pain
and breathe it like an element.

Pain is, as Chasin observes, elemental in the process of childbirth. Just as pain and death are inseparable, so too are pain and birth. A dense layer of suffering envelops our corporeal world, and all souls wishing to enter or leave must push their way through it at their own peril.

Curiously, few people question the wisdom of using medical technology to cause painless death, yet many question the wisdom of using the same technology to achieve painless birth. Society considers the great number of cancer patients who die in great pain as an abject failure of the modern physician, yet each day women around the globe scream and pant their way through hours of unending labor rather than seek artificial pain relief. I find this odd. Why reject the natural agonies of cancer and embrace the natural agonies of childbirth? True, labor pain is brief, at most a day or two in duration, but it's also extreme. In quantitative ratings of pain severity, the pain of a first labor exceeds cancer pain by a considerable margin and falls just shy of the pain of limb amputation sans anesthesia. Why endure such torment willingly? No rational person would want to have a leg cut off without benefit of modern painkilling technique, yet thousands of women pay money to learn how to avoid anesthesia during childbirth. The pain of birth is no different from any other pain...or is it?

The introduction of general anesthesia into the birthing process in 1847 by James Young Simpson touched off a firestorm of controversy that burns to the present day. One camp argues that birth should be as painless as possible, even if relief comes in the form of drugs, nerve blocks, even general anesthesia; the opposing camp contends that childbirth should be free of all undue medical interference despite the great suffering such freedom imposes on the mother. What drives this strange controversy? Is the resistance to pharmacologic pain control during the birthing process a cultural phenomenon, akin to the New Age fads of crystal energy and pyramid power, or does the desire for natural birth derive from some primitive neurological urge to feel the pain of creation? Scholars have been struggling to decipher the strange symbiosis between pain and the birthing process for centuries. They've made progress, but mysteries surrounding the psychology and physiology of childbirth pain still abound.

The trauma required for the creation of new life varies widely in the biological realm. The most primitive cellular life-forms, including protozoans, fungi, and bacteria, literally rip themselves in two. Oak trees, on the other hand, silently drop their acorns to the ground. Fish, birds, reptiles, amphibians, and a few mammal species (for example, the platypus) lay eggs, a comparatively painless process as far as we can judge. Viruses don't even bother with their own reproduction, choosing instead to have other living things do it for them.

Most mammals, however, resort to the ancient single-cell strategy of tearing their bodies apart. Creating a large, complex mammal like the human infant from a single ovum is an arduous and nutritionally demanding process—too demanding to occur independent of the mother's body in some self-contained egg. Pea-brained chickens may be grown in this way; building a brainy human in like fashion would require so much nutrient yolk that the resulting egg would be the size of a small automobile.

Most fetal mammals must therefore stay tethered to their

mother's bloodstream throughout development. So intertwined are their circulatory systems that mother and child function as one organism until the moment of separation. Once gestation is complete, the mother's body extrudes the child and their mutual bond divides in a torrent of fluid and blood. Our warm and gentle feelings about childbirth are misguided. In humans, the process is a thing of terror and violence. A woman's genitals and pelvic floor stretch to the breaking point and beyond. The vagina and rectum can be torn irreparably, the pelvic bones separated, the bladder smashed. The muscular uterus spasms with such vehemence that the child can be ejected like a missile. The first child I delivered as a medical student hit me in the chest and almost knocked the wind out of me (the child, fortunately, was unharmed). There is little gentle about this process.

Comedienne Joan Rivers once said that the stretching of genital skin needed to yield a baby can be simulated by grabbing the lower lip and yanking it over the top of the head. She meant to be funny, but her analogy actually understates the situation. Given these rapid distortions of anatomy, it's no wonder labor and delivery are so painful, particularly for first-time mothers. Nevertheless, it remains more than a little mysterious that a process so essential to the procreation of our species should be such a fearful and agonizing experience.

As I've argued previously, natural selection doesn't bother with mercy unless it facilitates our survival and procreation. Nature doesn't protect us against cancer pain because cancer isn't a threat to our species. There's been no evolutionary impetus to produce painless cancers. In the case of childbirth, however, mercy should prevail since there's a very good Darwinian impetus for painless childbirth: the more childbirth hurts, the less inclined mothers will be to have children. This is especially true for human beings. Thanks to our huge brains, we have an excellent memory for pain and can devise complex strategies to avoid it.

In fact, we're so intelligent that we can avoid painful experiences we've seen but haven't personally experienced. Cows, for example, won't be put off by a barbed-wire fence simply because they've witnessed other cows getting tangled in it. They have to experience the pain firsthand. But in humans, watching a single painful childbirth might frighten an entire community of women out of bearing children. This isn't a theoretical concern. I have known more than one woman who opted not to have a child because of their fear of childbirth, and this is in the age of anesthesia. One can only imagine the inhibitory fear of childbirth in the preanesthetic era.

Thus, it seems in our best interest as a species for our childbirth to be a pleasurable experience. After all, isn't that why sexual intercourse feels so good, to encourage us to make babies? Why gratify us at one end of gestation and torture us at the other? Yet nature shows women no mercy during childbirth.

Why?

I suspect that this lack of mercy wasn't intentional. There must have been great evolutionary pressures to reduce the misery of childbirth, but perhaps there wasn't enough time to do so. Consider the case of spinal disc disorders. As discussed previously, our rapid conversion from small-headed quadripeds to big-headed bipeds forced our spines to do things they weren't designed to do. The basic architecture of vertebrates evolved over hundreds of millions of years and was built to carry weight evenly distributed over a horizontal posture. In less than a million years, the same design was subsequently forced upright and, even worse, made to carry a mammoth head perched at its apex. With insufficient time to adapt the old spinal technology to this new posture, evolution sentenced us to the miseries of spinal pain.

It was a calculated trade-off: evolution balanced the benefits of unencumbered forelimbs against the sporadic incapacity produced by failing spines. The fact that our planet currently crawls with countless human bodies proves that this trade-off was worthwhile. Given another hundred million years, nature might yet work out the kinks in our spines, but, until then, we're stuck with jerry-rigged technology that has yet to keep pace with the demands placed on it.

Painful childbirth is a similar casualty of humankind's rapid entrance onto biology's stage. Our large head size evolved over an even shorter period of time than our erect posture. We know, for example, that the earliest bipeds still looked like pinheads compared to modern humans. As this rapid cranial expansion took place, female pelvic anatomy, like the spine, was confronted with the difficult task of adapting old technology to radical new uses. A birth canal designed to pass large litters of small, streamlined animals now had to accommodate the passage of one or two bulbous-headed progeny. It could be done, of course, but it was going to hurt. There wasn't much that natural selection could do to prevent the escalation of childbirth pain caused by the expanding human head, certainly not in a scant fifty thousand generations. The only feasible ways to do this would be to give women a massive pelvis or to render the pelvis and genitals permanently anesthetic. Neither would be tenable. Creating permanently insensate genitals or an outsized pelvis simply to ameliorate a half dozen transiently painful experiences didn't make survival sense. As such, women are stuck with their painful

ordeal, at least until natural selection comes up with a better solution in another million years or so.

The extreme stress placed on the birth canal during the passage of a human fetus has another unfortunate consequence:
Childbirth became dangerous. Death during labor and delivery is
relatively rare in all animals save humans. Prior to the advent of
modern obstetrics, childbirth claimed the lives of three out of
every hundred laboring mothers. Over multiple births, mothers
in the premodern era had a significant lifetime risk of death, although our prodigious survival proves that our big heads were
worth the risk.

Jared Diamond, in his book *The Third Chimpanzee,* postulates
that the great dangers of human childbirth account for another
misery unique to human females: menopause. Human females
are fertile for about thirty years—less than one half of their natural life spans. While fertility declines somewhat with age in all
mammals, including human men, only human women shut down
their reproductive systems completely many years before they
die. Diamond considers menopause a protective reflex. Women
older than fifty may not be capable of withstanding childbirth.
Moreover, the long period of a human child's vulnerability makes
a mother's survival essential to the survival of her children. In
short, she's simply too valuable to risk in never-ending cycles of
pregnancy and childbirth. The human reproductive system allows each woman a limited opportunity to have children and then
shields her from further risk. The relative period of infertility
that occurs when new mothers are breastfeeding also protects the
new infant from quickly losing a mother to a new pregnancy.

As I watched my wife strain to expel my daughter that night,
I wasn't concerned about the survival of my species, only about
her survival and the survival of our daughter. My wife in her bed

and me in my chair, we both were witness to the steep price demanded by nature for the honor of being Homo sapiens— thinking man.

⇒

Childbirth pain isn't entirely unique to humans. The cramping of uterine contractions and the painful dilation of cervix and vagina affects most mammals, except, perhaps, the egg-laying platypus and marsupials like the kangaroo, which gives birth to tiny fetuses that then crawl into the mother's pouch to complete their final gestation. Any veterinarian can relate tales of difficult labors in horses, cows, and other beasts. Nevertheless, severe and frequent birthing pains seem limited to primates like us. In a 1985 study of pregnant monkeys and apes, over three quarters of laboring mothers exhibited signs of severe distress, including grimacing and writhing during labor and crying out during delivery, suggesting that our primate cousins also suffer during childbirth. Since we have the largest heads of any primates, our females suffer the most.

⇒

Because the size of our heads makes a painful childbirth unavoidable, nature came up with three tricks to compensate for the chilling effect that childbirth pain might exert on human reproductive behaviors. The first trick has already been mentioned: the joy of sex. Although we have a long memory for pain, we're also notorious for doing fun things despite the sorry consequences that will follow later. We get drunk fully aware of the hangover awaiting us the next day. We play that yearly volleyball game at the family reunion even though we know we won't be able to move for three days. A close friend of mine is allergic to shrimp, but he enjoys the crustaceans so much he still eats them and accepts that he will be sicker than a dog hours later. Since sex comes ahead of shrimp on the average person's "to do" list, it's no wonder that the consequences of childbirth may have little impact on the rate of impregnation.

The second trick is biochemical. Late in pregnancy the rising levels of endogenous narcotic substances known as endorphins increase the expectant mother's tolerance of pain. The hormone relaxin also softens the pelvic tissues, permitting easier deformation of the pelvic outlet during birth. How much these hormones increase the mother's actual comfort is debatable, but these changes show that the female body is trying to ameliorate the pain as best it can.

The final trick is much sneakier: silent ovulation. A female is fertile for only a few days following the release of a fresh ovum. In most mammals, the female undergoes visible changes in appearance and behavior during her fertile window. She becomes sexually aggressive and indiscriminant in her mating; her genitals may swell or change color and she may emit odors signaling her fertility. The human female, save for feeling an occasional mild pain caused by the rupture of a ripe ovarian follicle, remains oblivious to her ovulation. In fact, so silent is human ovulation that the timing of ovum release relative to the menstrual cycle wasn't deciphered by endocrinologists until 1930. Studies of sexual intercourse frequency during the menstrual cycle further suggest that couples have no clear knowledge of the time of maximum fertility; thus, there appears to be no covert signs of ovulation either—no subliminal body language, no chemical cues.

In *The Third Chimpanzee*, Diamond postulates that silent ovulation, like menopause, is also a biological phenomenon mandated by our hazardous and painful births. If ovulation were obvious, Diamond's argument goes, clever women would quickly learn to avoid intercourse during their fertile period, thereby enjoying the pleasures of sex without the consequences of pregnancy and childbirth. Silent ovulation makes this natural birth control impossible.

In addition to biological adaptations like pleasurable intercourse and silent ovulation, we have also developed cultural methods for hiding the pain of childbirth from impressionable young females. In his controversial study of human behavior, *The Naked Ape*, zoologist Desmond Morris popularized the idea that cultural practices often derive from biological necessity. In the spirit of Morris, I propose that childbirth rituals reflect the biological necessity of minimizing the negative impact of childbirth pain. Women throughout history and in diverse societies often sought to give birth alone or with the aid of older (and often postmenopausal) women. Granted, solitary birth is not uncommon among mammals, but humans are exquisitely social beings who usually seek out the sympathy of others in times of acute distress. Although solitude also makes good hygienic sense, it also keeps the birthing experience "in the closet." Childless women can't fear what they don't know.

In crowded civilizations like Japan where isolation is nearly impossible, women developed an immense stoicism during childbirth. This stoicism gave rise to the myth that childbirth pain itself is a modern cultural phenomenon. Early proponents of "natural childbirth" (including Grantly Dick-Read, the obstetrician who coined the phrase in the 1930s) believed that "primitive" cultures (more correctly, "nonwhite" cultures) were immune to labor pain entirely. "Primitives," as such women were called, simply dropped their children in the fields as effortlessly as having a bowel movement. "The primitive," Dick-Read wrote in his 1933 monograph "Natural Childbirth," "knows that she will have little trouble when her child is born."

In Dick-Read's paradigm, childbirth pain is an invention of pampered, out-of-shape white Europeans and could be cured by stripping them of their high society softheadedness. If they could only emulate their brown and yellow sisters, things would go easier for them. This sounds a tad racist, and it is. But then, there's more than a little racism in the early theories of childbirth pain. Dick-Read felt that "primitives" (a definition that included some fairly advanced cultures) don't think about their labors and so develop no fear and experience no tension or pain. The unstated implication is that these women are too simpleminded to be frightened or hurt by anything. Some early authors even considered childbirth pain the bane of women who mate outside of their "own kind." George Engelmann, in his excellent history of obstetrics published in 1882, writes that labor pain is worse when a woman is trying to deliver a "half-breed," perhaps, he speculates, because the size and shape of the child doesn't mesh with her pelvic anatomy.

In the final analysis, the idea that childbirth pain is a product of modern civilization is, in a word, hogwash. In Genesis, a document thousands of years old, God warns the fallen Eve that she and her descendants will give birth in pain. The Bible later favorably compares the courage of women in labor to the courage of men in battle. Clearly, ancient cultures were well aware of child-birth's difficulties. In 1945 C. S. Ford studied the pain of birth in sixty-four so-called "primitive" cultures and concluded that "the popular impression of childbirth in primitive societies as painless and easy is definitely contraindicated in our cases. As a matter of fact, it is often prolonged and painful."

Although pain itself isn't influenced by culture, expression of pain clearly depends upon cultural biases. A Japanese woman may display no outward signs of discomfort during labor, but when asked to fill out a questionnaire afterward, she will rate pain severity the same as women of European descent. Childbirth stoicism in crowded civilizations may serve the same purpose that solitude does in more rural societies, namely, to protect impressionable young women from learning the truth about labor's trials and tribulations. If you can't scream where no one hears you, don't scream at all.

If this all seems far-fetched, remember that very small influences on reproductive behavior can cause significant perturbations in a species over thousands of generations. Had labor been treated as a public event throughout our history, there's little doubt certain females would be put off by the experience. This might have introduced an undesirable selection bias into the human genome. We don't know what common traits the birth-aversive women might have shared, traits that would have been selected out of the general population.

Could the simple acts of holding one's tongue during uterine contractions or going alone into the bushes to deliver a child have had any great impact on our species? Maybe not. But then, the re-production of animals often hinges on seemingly silly things like the performance of an intricate dance, the sweetness of a song, or the coloration of a tail feather. Minuscule variations in mating behaviors can alter interbreeding in a way that redirects the course of the species' development.

✦

Which brings us back to the controversy between the two camps, one favoring medical pain control and the other a natural labor and delivery. If biological factors might drive behaviors like stoicism and isolation during birthing, could such factors also drive a woman's yearning to give birth the old-fashioned way, under her own control and in her own blessed pain?

So far I've only mentioned the negative aspects of labor pain. Like other forms of pain, the pain of childbirth may be a double-edged sword, possessing both good and bad aspects. Women who have endured a particularly grueling labor may question whether there was any kernel of "good" in the experience, but labor pain may indeed serve a purpose.

Return to the title of my introduction: "The Megaphone of God." For the purposes of this discussion, childbirth pain may be better termed the Megaphone of Baby. After my wife had her epidural, the labor slowed. Without the driving effect of pain, a woman's mental focus on the urgent task at hand may wander. Labor is a dangerous time. With each uterine contraction, the blood flow through the placenta becomes compromised. As the baby descends into the birth canal, the head is deformed, literally squashed. None of these derangements has any lasting consequences provided they don't go on too long. Escalating pain forces the mother to pay attention and drive the event to completion as quickly as possible.

Tribes in northern Russia had a curious custom. During difficult labors, husband and wife had to discuss details of their

sexual affairs with others. This unpleasantness presumably stim-
ulated both parties to keep the labor, and conversation, as short as
possible. Pain may play the same role: speed. The mother knows
what she must do to end the pain—deliver the baby. Like the
caller on a rowing team, the pain yells through its megaphone for
her to keep stroking toward the finish line.

This isn't just idle speculation on my part. The need for a
rapid labor and the role that pain plays in hurrying labor along
have been known for centuries. Some cultures took to threatening or frightening the baby hurriedly out of the womb. The
Alaskan poem at the beginning of this chapter speaks of terrifying the child, a common theme. Klamath Indian mothers told
their infants that a rattlesnake was crawling into the womb to bite
them if they didn't come out. Pahute mothers fasted during the
final month of gestation in the belief that the child could be
starved out, like starving a woodchuck from its den.

Other cultures sought to increase a mother's pain in hopes of
shortening labor. Russians of northern Asia used herbs believed
to heighten pain sensitivity, while the Kazak of central Asia were
more brutal: they held a woman's hand to a fire to keep labor
moving. In the Philippines midwives placed wooden planks
across the woman's abdomen and applied direct pressure to the
womb. Notice that none of these maneuvers took the mother's
comfort into consideration. Speed, not pain control, was the goal.

Plant remedies were common, but once again they were used
for enhancing speed, not comfort. The ancient Mexicans routinely used the civapacthi plant to stimulate uterine contractions,
much as modern obstetricians use the uterine stimulant oxytocin.
A variety of other oxytocin-like herbs been employed throughout the world. Some cultures used plants in a mechanical fashion
by inserting dry leaves into the cervix. As the leaves soaked up

uterine secretions, they expanded and dilated the cervix, again speeding labor.

With the advent of general anesthesia in the last century, physicians could now eliminate the pain of labor entirely. In doing so, they also slowed labor. This spurred the creation of a new device: the forceps, a pair of spoonlike metal instruments that allowed the obstetrician to reach into the birth canal and yank out the recalcitrant child. They did the job, but not without problems. Babies are designed to be pushed out of the vagina, not pulled out. Improperly or aggressively used, forceps could fracture the skull, harm the facial nerves (causing facial paralysis), even break the poor child's neck. Surely this isn't how nature intended children to be born—rudely pulled from a sedated or unconscious mother.

The obvious absurdity of this form of delivery helped spur a return to natural birthing practices in the middle part of this century. However, the man most responsible for popularizing natural childbirth, Grantly Dick-Read, advocated anesthesia-free birth for stranger reasons. In his 1944 book *Childbirth without Fear,* Dick-Read wrote: "The pain of labor, and its initiating cause, fear, extend their evil influence into the very roots of our social structure. They corrupt the minds and bodies of successive generations and bring distress and calamity where happiness and prosperity are the reward of a simple physiological performance." Dick-Read felt that natural childbirth created a primal force he called "motherlove," which could, in proper quantity, cure all the world's ills, from poverty to disease. He described his work as "no longer an obstetric practice only, but a mission—no longer a pursuit, but a calling."

Dick-Read and the other major advocate of natural birth, Paris obstetrician Fernand Lamaze (who imported the Pavlovian

methods of childbirth used in the Soviet Union), didn't see pain
as a necessary force that could be controlled and harnessed for
the good of mother and child, but viewed pain instead as an evil
interloper, something that by rights didn't belong in the birthing
process at all. Dick-Read saw labor pain as a manifestation of fear
alone, with no physiological role whatsoever. Those who advocate natural childbirth today must remember that Dick-Read's
original intent was not the *management* of labor pain, but the
abolition of labor pain. In Dick-Read's paradigm, labor pain
shouldn't exist at all.

Dick-Read's mystic outlook no doubt traces back to the origins of his beliefs about pain and the mind. During trench
warfare of World War I, a shell-shocked Dick-Read learned his
Eastern relaxation techniques from an Indian noncommissioned
officer. Eventually he came to think of his methods as capable of
changing world history; by restoring childbirth to its pristine,
natural state, Dick-Read could purge the world of evil. Critics
questioned why women had to spend so much time learning "natural" techniques like the Dick-Read and Lamaze methods when
"natural childbirth" should be so instinctive.

And Dick-Read had numerous critics to be sure, including
competitor Lamaze. He gave abuse out as quickly as it came in,
too, dismissing Lamaze's methods as just another attempt by the
Russians to take credit for everything, even Shakespeare. One of
his biggest foes was the National Birthday Trust Fund, or NBTF,
a private organization in his native England that advocated the
use of anesthesia in childbirth and raised money to allow poor
women to have the same access to medically assisted births as
rich women enjoyed. The NBTF funded research into safer anesthetic techniques, taught midwives how to administer home anesthesia, successfully lobbied the British Parliament to repeal laws

against the administration of anesthesia by midwives, and even distributed chloroform ampules for that purpose. Thanks to the NBTF, labor pain became politicized, a form of class warfare. Poor women suffered because they were poor. The NBTF wanted all women to have the "Princess drugs," as they called the narcotics given to Princess (now Queen) Elizabeth during her delivery of Prince Charles.

Gradually, however, natural birth advocates began to turn the tide. Dick-Read even got an endorsement from Pope Pius XII, who penned an encyclical about childbirth in 1957. Although any method of alleviating childbirth pain may be contrary to divine intent, mused the pope, he found nothing in Catholic doctrine prohibiting the use of Dick-Read's or Lamaze's methods. The Pope preferred Dick-Read's "English" approach, feeling it allowed a more "Christian Delivery" than Lamaze's "Russian" method. It was hard to imagine anything Christian emanating from the Soviet Union in the 1950s, a fact not lost on the Holy Father. The Pope awarded Dick-Read a silver medal for his work, apparently overlooking the physician's earlier claim that Christianity was one of the biggest sources of unnatural labor pain in the first place.

Although the teachings of men like Grantly Dick-Read were often misguided, their message has validity. Putting women to sleep and pulling out their babies with makeshift barbecue tongs had serious drawbacks. Moreover, their assertion that women can be prepared mentally and physically for the rigors of childbirth in such a way that it becomes a tolerable and satisfying experience for them, even without drugs or needles, has also proven correct. For our second child, my wife and I completed full Lamaze training, and that labor went smoothly and without anesthetic help. Of course, second children tend to be easier than the first, but I was convinced that the preparation we received was indispensable. Maybe it was just a mental thing—but then, pain is often just a mental thing. Even my chair felt more comfortable.

The natural route shouldn't be carried to extremes. Techniques such as epidural anesthesia, caudal blocks, and even cesarean section may be necessary to provide a comfortable and safe delivery. Each case must be handled individually, and no woman should feel guilty about how she performs during labor. She should use whatever tools she has at her disposal to survive the experience unscathed. The only option my immigrant grandmother had was natural childbirth, and it yielded her a son paralyzed and brain-injured by a botched home delivery.

There's one other reproductive pain women endure: menstruation. Menstruation is truly a uniquely human pain—I can find no reference to menstrual discomfort in other animals. As in the case of childbirth, menstrual cramps have been dismissed as a modern manifestation, the complaining of weak women. Once again, the historical record contradicts this. The Koran calls menstruation "a hurt" and that's about as succinct a description as any. The ancient physician and anatomist Galen notes the pain of menstruation; he postulated that women menstruate because they are so idle most of the time they have to shed the excess sweat and blood that men routinely work off. I doubt Galen makes the National Organization for Women's top ten list of admired men.

The pain derives from the uterine spasms and hormonal surges that occur normally during the monthly menstrual cycle. These symptoms may, like migraine, help steer sexual intercourse to the middle part of the cycle, where fertility is greatest. If so, then add menstruation to the list of things we can blame on our big heads.

Stop and consider all of the possible consequences of our outsized brains. It certainly makes childbirth hazardous and painful, so hazardous that the female reproductive period must be abruptly terminated (menopause). Painful childbirth, in turn, could also account for the pleasurable sensation of intercourse, and explain why our ovulation is so silent—we have to be teased or duped into going through the experience of childbirth. This silent ovulation means we have no period of heat like animals, so we have to be nudged into having sexual intercourse at the right time. Since the days before, during, and after menstruation are precisely the wrong time, women suffer a variety of ailments— migraines, cramps, mood swings—that make intercourse the last thing on their minds. We also developed social taboos concerning sex and menstruation, in some cultures to the point of labeling menstruating women unclean, unholy, even dangerous. The bumper sticker that reads "I have PMS and a gun, any questions?" shows that the "dangerous" label still lingers.

Dysmenorrhea—incapacitating menstrual cramps—and other chronic pelvic pain in women (including pain from endometriosis, sexually transmitted illnesses, and pelvic pain of unknown origin) exact an alarming toll on society, considering that these are nonlethal conditions. A study in the United Kingdom found that nearly 1 percent of all health care dollars spent in 1991 went toward menstrual disorders and female pelvic pain. Including lost time from work, dysmenorrhea is a billion-dollar problem.

Dysmenorrhea usually responds well to oral contraceptives used in conjunction with over-the-counter analgesics. But there is no cure for this condition, which carries the appropriate nickname "the curse."

⇌

While reading about birth customs, I was most impressed by one practiced by the Aztecs of ancient Mexico. An Aztec woman who died in labor was buried with full military honors as a war hero and her family granted a pension. The Aztecs saw birth as "the woman's war" and, having seen it myself many times, I agree. It represents a woman's life-and-death struggle with her child, herself, and her species. For my brain to be large enough to write these pages, my mother and her mother before her had to wage that war. In birth, we see a courage equal to that shown by Christ in Gethsemane, the courage to face an almost unbearable ordeal simply because it is what must be done. The Aztecs practiced human sacrifice and played soccer with human heads, but their reverence for women should be a model for those of us who live in a more "enlightened" age.

6 THE HORROR

The joints of thy thighs are like jewels,
the work of the hands of a cunning workman.

—Song of Solomon 7:1

When seeing new patients in my office, I try guessing what's wrong with them using clues derived from their appearance and mannerisms. I later compare my conclusions to patient profiles provided by their referring physicians. Pretending to be Sherlock Holmes, I enjoy striding about the clinic wearing my imaginary deerstalker cap, deducing the patient's disease from the shape of the fingernails or the posture of the spine. Holmes buffs will see nothing odd in a surgeon comparing himself to the legendary Baker Street sleuth; after all, Holmes himself was based, at least partially, on a real-life surgeon, Dr. Joseph Bell, an early mentor of the young Conan Doyle. Legend has it that Bell could tell where a patient lived by the color of the dust on his boots.

Unfortunately, I didn't need any of my Holmesian powers to deduce what was ailing Clara. She sat hunched in her wheelchair, her bony hands misshapen to the point of uselessness. The extreme distortion of her fingers could be caused by only one disease: rheumatoid arthritis, or RA. The phrase comes from the

Greek word *arthron* for "joint" and *rheumos,* meaning "flux" (I don't know what the word *flux* has to do with rheumatic diseases, but that's the origin of the word).

The rosy roundness of her face posed a stark contrast to the sticklike arms and legs—no doubt she had been on steroids for many years. Peering through a crack in the exam room door, I watched how her every move was steeped in pain. She winced as she adjusted her stiff frame in the seat, gasping softly as she repositioned her arthritic hands on the wheelchair's vinyl armrests.

Even if she hadn't been wearing that bulky cervical collar, I could easily guess why she had come to see me. There is but a single reason a lifelong RA sufferer seeks the advice of a neurosurgeon: her disease now attacked the joints in her neck and distorted the alignment of the vertebrae, just as it had distorted her fingers. As RA erodes the supporting pillars of the cervical spine, the uppermost vertebra slowly moves forward and will slice the spinal cord in two if left unchecked. Early anatomists called the first vertebra Atlas because it supports the weight of the head like Atlas supporting the weight of the world. In RA, Atlas, standing astride two diseased neck joints, begins to lose his footing and the head topples inexorably forward.

Spinal cord injury at the level of Atlas causes a swift death. It's the preferred injury of merciful hangmen. The relentless migration of the spine can only be halted by surgically bonding Atlas to one of the adjacent vertebra using metal wires or bone screws. It's a brutal therapy to be sure, particularly in elderly patients debilitated by years of disease and the ravaging effects of powerful drugs, but no easier alternative exists. The disease that had tortured Clara for her entire adult life now sought to finish her off. (Not if I could help it, of course.)

What causes RA? What makes the joints of otherwise healthy

people swell, throb, and contort until they fuse into immobile masses of bone? While the world frets about deadly diseases, nonlethal conditions like RA are left to rob us of more productive years than AIDS and cancer combined.

Unlike the recently evolved miseries of disc disease and childbirth, RA's roots lie in the distant past. Clara's illness started over forty years ago, but the mechanisms responsible for it began hundreds of millions of years before that, during a time when skeletons and joints didn't even exist.

To understand Clara's disease, we must go all the way back to the primal origin of large multicellular creatures like ourselves. Although we think of bodies as single organisms, they are, in fact, enormous colonies of individual cells. We are giant ant farms, social ensembles consisting of about 10 trillion living, breathing beings. And, just as an ant farm employs individuals adapted to special purposes—workers, warriors, queens, food handlers— our cells have adapted to their own unique roles as nerve cells, muscle cells, blood cells, and so on.

Like the origin of life itself, the origin of the social integration of free-living cells into multicellular organisms took place long before the fossil record, making it impossible to know exactly how or when this seminal event took place. We do know that at some point in our history, a few enterprising cells decided that they would be better off joining forces rather than continuing to go it alone. These cells merged into the first multicellular organisms and began sharing the rent, so to speak.

At first these larger organisms behaved like 1960s communes: everyone was welcome and the more the groovier. As they became larger and more formally organized, however, colonies grew more selective, even xenophobic. Outsiders were no longer tolerated. Like survivors crowding onto a full lifeboat, intruder cells could swamp the whole colony and had to be kept out or, if they couldn't take a hint, killed outright. The concept of "us versus them" was born—and persists to this day in the form of organ rejection and gated neighborhoods. We reject new livers and new neighbors for the same reason that ancient organisms turned away new additions to their colonies: Whatever isn't "us" must be bad. Chauvinism is in our blood. Literally.

To keep their neighborhoods pure, primitive organisms had to devise ways of delineating and enforcing their newly established borders. The first step was to define exactly what constituted "us" and what constituted "them." To this end, cells deployed protein markers on their outer surfaces to prove that they belonged to a given cell colony, just as modern soldiers use different uniforms to identify their allegiance and street thugs use special clothing to proclaim their membership in a gang. Soon each multicellular organism had a unique protein uniform. If a new cell entering the colony wore a friendly uniform, it was welcome; if not, it was killed. The battle lines were drawn.

Uniforms and borders don't mean much, though, without armed enforcement. All living communities, even the most primitive, use military force to maintain their integrity. In nature, taking things through violence is fair game and protecting what's yours through violence becomes mandatory. Termites and ants have a soldier caste, bees and wasps equip their workers with weapons, and humans build armies. The most rudimentary organisms developed enforcer cells, little versions of Dirty Harry assigned to terminate with extreme prejudice any cells that didn't wear the appropriate uniform. The first cellular enforcers devised a simple fighting strategy: they simply crawled up to foreign cells and ate them, a trick known as phagocytosis, from the Greek words *phagos,* "to eat," and *cytos,* "cell." (Perhaps Hannibal Lecter makes a more fitting movie analogy here than Dirty Harry Callahan.)

In the microscopic world, phagocytosis is the most fundamental killing tool, analogous to shooting or blowing things up in the military. Although we now use lasers and computers to guide our bombs, the military's goal hasn't changed a great deal since the days of Napoléon: find the enemy and blow them to bits. Likewise, although mammals now use advanced weapons like antibodies (the smart bombs of biology), sooner or later an invader, whether a bacterium or a transplanted heart, will be eaten.

The first tiny organisms didn't need an organized military. They randomly deployed their enforcer cells like bouncers in a bar. The enforcers simply waited and watched, ready to eject any party crashers on a moment's notice. Very large organisms like us, on the other hand, must use a different form of military deployment. We bivouac our enforcers in centralized locations, like the lymph nodes and spleen, then dispatch them in great hordes through the bloodstream to potential trouble spots.

To coordinate the large-scale mobilization of enforcer cells, animals developed complex chemical signals that would alert enforcers as to when and where a foreign invasion took place. Suppose a tree branch lacerates an animal's skin and contaminates the wound with dirt and bacteria. The contaminated tissues emit a cry for help, releasing molecules called cytokines (from the Greek *cytos,* "cell," and *kinesis,* "to set in motion"). Cytokines are potent hormones that trigger a cascade of events designed to repel any foreign invasion.

Immediately after an invasion, arteries feeding the point of entry dilate, increasing the local blood supply and causing the wound to redden and grow warm. Next the same blood vessels spring leaks, opening large holes in their walls to allow arriving enforcer cells to squeeze into surrounding tissues, where they begin their search-and-destroy patrols. In addition to allowing the enforcers to exit the bloodstream, leaky blood vessels also permit the blood's liquid serum to escape as well. The wound becomes swollen and boggy. Escaping serum turns to clot, welding the wound closed and reducing the risk of further contamination.

The cytokines attract ever-increasing numbers of enforcer cells (what we now call white blood cells). The cells descend on the wound like flies to honey and gorge themselves on bacterial invaders until they themselves die; the liquefying white cells and their consumed prey soon fill the area with a thick white soup that wells up and drains from the body in the form of pus. As the battle between "us" and "them" rages, the cytokines irritate surrounding nerve endings, making the injured area terribly painful. This forces a wounded animal to rest the damaged part until any continued threat of invasion has passed. Reduced bodily movement limits the spread of contagion and hastens the permanent sealing of the wound with scar tissue.

This choreographed series of cytokine-orchestrated events, which starts at the moment of injury and lasts for several days or longer, is the most ancient form of biological defense known and has a familiar name: inflammation.

＊

Physicians of antiquity knew all about inflammation. The oldest known medical textbook, the Edwin Smith papyrus penned by Egyptian healers seventeen centuries before the birth of Christ, called the body's reaction to injury "*shememet*." The word *shememet* is always followed by a hieroglyph for "fire" to symbolize the redness and heat that are the hallmarks of acute inflammation. A thousand years after the papyrus appeared, Greek physician Hippocrates called inflammation "*phlegmone*," which loosely translates as "the burning thing." In the first century A.D., Roman author Cornelius Celsus provided a succinct Latin description of inflammation that is taught to medical students even today: *Rubor et tumor cum calore et dolore* (Redness and swelling with heat and pain).

The modern study of inflammation began with pathologist Julius Cohnheim in the 1860s. Cohnheim placed caustic substances on the tongues of live frogs and studied the resulting inflammatory changes under a microscope. Because frog tongues are thin and transparent, Cohnheim could directly observe the progressive leakiness and dilation of small arteries together with the ensuing aggregation of white cells caused by irritating toxins. Given the rudimentary state of biochemistry at that time, Cohnheim could make no guess as to what initiated these events.

In the 1920s Sir Thomas Lewis of London postulated that an innate hormone triggered inflammation, but his astute speculation wasn't tested until the 1950s. Subsequent research proved Sir Thomas was correct, or partly correct. Inflammation isn't triggered by one substance as Sir Thomas presumed, but by hundreds of different cytokines merging into a hormonal symphony, chemical music composed millions of years ago. Unique cytokines mediate each phase of the inflammatory process—the arterial dilation, the vessel leakiness, the summoning of white cells, the production of pain.

The hormonal control of inflammation has more than aca-
demic importance. Most known "anti-inflammatory" drugs, from
the oldest (aspirin) to the newest (COX-2 inhibitors), disrupt the
cytokine symphony in some fashion. Our eventual conquest of
inflammatory diseases like RA requires the intimate understanding of all chemical signals responsible for that ancient process we
call inflammation.

➤

I could easily find the four cardinal signs of Celsus in Clara.
Her acutely inflamed right knee was pink and warm to the touch;
it was also quite swollen and exquisitely tender. Unlike bland
osteoarthritis, which affects us all after the age of forty-five, RA is
an inflammatory arthritis that can strike at any age. If I aspirated
Clara's knee joint with a needle and syringe, I would find the
same purulent broth that wells up in a dirty wound. But therein
lies the great mystery of RA. If inflammation evolved as a way of
repelling invaders like bacteria, why does it occur inside sterile
knees, necks, and fingers of RA sufferers? Clara's knee had no
open wound and never did; there were no bacteria to be repelled
inside her joints, at least not anymore, and no foreign tissues to
reject, no soil to flush out in a river of pus. So what match ignites
the flame of inflammation in the joints of RA victims, condemn-
ing them to lifetimes of *rubor, calore, tumor,* and, most terribly,
dolor?

Bacterial infections can indeed cause an inflammatory arthritis similar to RA (gonorrhea is a common cause of infectious
arthritis in men), but despite decades of searching, no bacterial
organisms have been reliably cultured out of RA joints. As we
will see, some as yet unknown infection may initiate RA, but what

keeps it going is something more sinister than simple infection. Something horrible, in fact.

The horror autotoxicus.

There *is* a foreign invader inside the joints of RA victims, but that invader proves not to be foreign at all. Amazingly, the white cells of RA patients aren't attacking bacteria inside the joints— they're attacking the joints themselves! Like a snake eating its own tail, the RA victim slowly consumes her own joints, mistaking them for foreign tissue and rejecting them as she would reject joints transplanted from another body. It's all a bad case of mistaken identity.

Our joints are lined with a filmy tissue known as synovium. Synovium produces an oily lubricating fluid very similar in consistency to egg white, hence the name *syn-ovium:* "with egg." Early in the course of the disease, synovial tissues of RA victims somehow end up wearing enemy uniforms. Precisely how this happens remains unknown. The disguised synovial cells get mistaken for spies and soon fall prey to their own white cells. The body's dutiful soldiers spend a lifetime gunning down their own joint tissues, finally killing the synovium. RA joints ultimately succumb to an unending barrage of friendly fire.

As the Bible says, our joints are truly jewels, the work of a master craftsman. Ultrasmooth cartilage, velvety synovium, and slick synovial fluid combine to create a device that glides ever so smoothly, painlessly. There's more friction between two pieces of wet ice than exists between the two bones gliding inside a healthy synovial joint. But under the inflammatory assault of RA, the synovium becomes thickened and scarred, the cartilage worn, the lubricating fluid thick and pasty. Cytokines within the joint activate nerve endings, making the joint even more sensitive to pain. The joint's clockwork precision falls victim to the continuous corrosion of inflammation, growing stiffer and more deformed. The pain only ends when, in the disease's final stages, the defeated synovium dies and the raw edges of denuded bone fuse together, obliterating the joint entirely, a process known as joint anklyosis (from the Greek *ankylos,* meaning "crooked").

Collectively, the body's white cell defenses are known as the immune system, from the Latin word *immunis,* meaning "exempt from taxation." A complex organ made up of billions of specialized white blood cells, the immune system is charged with knowing "us" from "them" (or, in the parlance of immunologists, distinguishing "self" from "nonself"). This remarkable ability of the immune system to ignore its own host while viciously destroying all invading pathogens is called tolerance.

Telling self from nonself—tolerance—is no easy task. Our bodies contain many millions of different molecules; the outside world of viruses, bacteria, and toxins contains billions more. How our immune system keeps all of these molecules neatly sorted into two bins—us and them—remains a deep mystery. In an instant my immune system must decide if a chunk of protein floating in my bloodstream is harmless debris from one of my own cells, or a hostile virus. If the immune system reacts too quickly to my own floating garbage, I would soon die of systemic inflammation; but if it reacts to a virus too slowly, I will surely die of infection.

Given the staggering number of dangerous proteins in the

biological realm, the immune system must act boldly and possess an encyclopedic memory. Unfortunately, faced with such a herculean task, even the most sophisticated of immune systems can occasionally become confused. Moreover, pathogens, such as bacteria, like to play tricks on our defenses, confusing our immune systems further. In other words, microbes like to "jam our radar" in order to gain unfettered access to our bodies. To see how this works, consider an analogy from the macroscopic world.

Being the overgrown adolescent that I am, I like to play video games at shopping malls. One popular game requires the player to shoot all enemy soldiers as they jump onscreen. The enemy soldiers, in turn, shoot back and try to kill the player. To keep the player guessing, the game occasionally throws a friendly soldier, hostage, or bystander on the screen; killing one of these innocents results in the instant loss of your hard-earned quarter. To make things even more difficult, the game's designers dress friendly characters in clothing similar to the uniforms of the enemy soldiers. In the heat of battle, inexperienced players end up whacking more friends than foes and losing their money quickly.

The game presents players with the same challenge that faces our immune systems: they must instantly distinguish friend from foe and then dispatch all foes without the slightest hesitation. Kill a friend—you lose. Wait too long to kill an enemy and he will shoot you—you lose again. The game's designers, who make more money if people lose quickly, try to confuse players by making friend and foe almost indistinguishable. Of course, they can't make friends and foes identical. If they did that, no one would waste their time and money playing the game in the first place.

In the great video game of life, bacteria and viruses are like game designers. They want us, the players, to lose occasionally and to this end have devised ways of confusing the immune system, hindering its ability to distinguish friend from foe. Microbes know that if they look too much like an enemy, our immune system will wipe them out easily and that's not good. If they look exactly like us, however, thus rendering our immunity impotent, humans would all soon die of contagion and that's not good, either. A parasite can't exist on a planet devoid of hosts. So microbes take the middle road, confusing our immune systems a little bit—but not too much.

Confronted with a daily battering of microbial smoke and mirrors, the immune system occasionally gets duped into attacking its own tissues like a video game player with an itchy trigger finger who shoots too many innocent bystanders. Pioneer immunologist Paul Virchow first proposed that a loss of immune "tolerance" for our own tissues might cause human illness. Writing at the turn of the century, Virchow called this condition the horror autotoxicus. He used the word *autotoxicus* because the disease was our innate toxicity directed against ourselves. He used the word *horror* because the situation was...well, horrible.

There's something obscene about committing violence against one's own flesh and blood. Emperor Caligula eating his own child, Buddhist priests committing self-immolation, the man who intentionally falls and breaks an arm in order to win a personal injury settlement, the teenager who pierces a tongue or nipple to gain peer acceptance, the circus freak who passes needles through his flesh or swallows swords—we see these acts as more than odd; they seem like crimes against nature, something horrible. Biology demands that we cling to life and guard our bodily integrity at all costs. To harm ourselves breaks some sacred oath carved deep in the marble of our genes.

Movie buffs will recognize the title of this chapter—"the horror, the horror"—as Marlon Brando's final words in *Apocalypse Now*. The more literary know that these words were first spoken by Kurtz, the fictional villain of Conrad's masterpiece *Heart of Darkness*. The movie is an updated adaptation of Conrad's novella. Both movie and novella probe the source of the world's evil, alias "the heart of darkness." Kurtz speaks his dying words as he peers deep into the heart of darkness and sees himself, a vision he finds horrible. The source of all evil, in Conrad's view, lives within ourselves. Therein, too, lies the horror of Virchow's horror autotoxicus. The corruption lies within ourselves, inside immune systems turned traitor. The organ sworn to protect Clara had decades ago turned on her and plopped her into a wheelchair. And it wasn't through with her yet.

Virchow's colorful moniker "horror autotoxicus" has today been replaced by a more clinical phrase: autoimmune disorder. RA is just one of many known autoimmune disorders. The immune system can be tricked into attacking almost any part of the body. My father contracted Hashimoto's thyroiditis several years ago—his thyroid gland has been totally consumed by an autoimmune inflammation and he must now subsist on thyroid pills. Myasthenia gravis, the progressive neurological disease that hampered legendary actor Laurence Olivier in his later life, is an autoimmune assault on the muscles; an autoimmune attack directed against the brain and spinal cord produces multiple sclerosis. Autoimmune destruction of the pancreas causes some cases of diabetes (in fact, some researchers feel that nearly all cases of juvenile diabetes are autoimmune in origin). Chronic viral hepatitis and AIDS may also involve some component of immune self-destruction.

Systemic lupus erythematosus, also called SLE or simply

lupus, is the most aggressive autoimmune disorder known. In lupus the immune system attacks everywhere at once—joints, kidneys, skin, brain, lungs, liver. The inflamed facial sores of lupus resemble wounds inflicted by some wild animal, hence the name (*lupus* is Latin for "wolf"). Lupus patients can suffer total shutdown of their kidneys, dementia, severe arthritis (equal to RA), and even heart failure as the immune system wreaks havoc in every nook and cranny of their bodies. The immune system of a lupus patient even attacks DNA, the very stuff of our creation. These immune systems are the Nazi skinheads of immunology, dysfunctional miscreants reduced to making obscene gestures at life itself.

❧

RA affects about one out of a hundred adults; a juvenile form exists, too. Most victims are women; in fact, many autoimmune disorders—including RA, lupus, Sjogren's syndrome, and the skin-hardening disease known as scleroderma—prefer females to males. The reason for this sexual disparity is unclear.

What causes an immune system to turn on its own host? The most likely culprit, as mentioned previously, is a microbial infection that throws sand in the immune system's eyes. Temporarily blinded, it begins attacking things indiscriminantly, killing the contagion but also vaccinating the host against her own tissues. We know that postinfectious autoimmunity does occur. For example, after certain influenza infections, we can mount an immune attack on our nerves, producing the autoimmune paralytic condition known as Guillain-Barré syndrome.

The infectious trigger for RA's autoimmunity, if one in fact exists, has yet to be found. Early researchers believed common tuberculosis initiated RA; although ultimately proven wrong, the tuberculous theory of RA produced a therapy still in common use today: gold injections. In 1890 Robert Koch, the father of modern microbiology (the study of bacteria and viruses), observed that gold salts inhibited the growth of tuberculosis bacilli in test tubes. In the 1920s, working on the mistaken belief that tuberculosis triggered RA, rheumatologists began administering gold injections to their patients with good results. We now know that gold therapy has nothing to do with tuberculosis but acts instead on the inflammatory process. Nevertheless, the story of gold therapy illustrates how good medicine can flow from erroneous theories.

Because autoimmunity may not begin until weeks after the acute infection clears, identifying the causative organism can be difficult. If we know what triggers diseases like RA, we might be able to stop them before they get started. This is an approach being used in the fight against diabetes. By studying the blood antibodies of juvenile diabetics in order to determine their past infections, researchers discovered that these patients share antibodies against the same cold virus, Coxsackie B; it's now believed that this virus is responsible for tricking thousands of children's bodies into attacking their own pancreatic tissues. Large-scale infant vaccinations against the virus might eliminate the disease entirely. Unfortunately, no similar scheme for RA exists. Even if it did, it would not help people like Clara who have already been rendered allergic to their own joints. For them, relief can only be found by silencing an immune system gone haywire.

Clara was first diagnosed with RA at the age of twenty-eight. Nevertheless, she married and raised two children, then went to work as a legal secretary until, at the age of fifty-one, her fingers grew too stiff to type at an acceptable speed. She retired to play golf but had to give that up after a few years because of the increasing pain in her back and knees. Surgeons replaced one knee with a prosthetic joint, but it never healed properly and she decided against any further joint replacements. Soon she was using a walker and then the wheelchair. During the year prior to her first visit to my office, Clara detected a progressive urgency of her bladder and a growing weakness in her upper arms. Her legs also began jumping at night, so much so that she had trouble sleeping. The jerking spasms would twist her inflamed hips and wake her every hour in a paroxysm of pain. Cervical spine X rays confirmed the growing deformity of her upper neck. The bladder disturbance and arm weakness, together with the leg spasticity, were cries for help, from her pinched spinal cord.

Despite years of health problems, Clara managed to wring many good things out of life. A family, a career, participation in sports. Even now, faced with another major surgery and a life spent in a wheelchair, she remained optimistic about her future. Much of her success in the face of adversity could be attributed to her own good cheer and strong will. But she had also had help, in the form of drugs like aspirin, gold, methotrexate, and, most recently, steroids. Without these medications, all the strong will and good cheer in the world would not have sufficed in the face of one of the most aggressive cases of RA I had ever seen.

Aspirin and aspirin-like compounds remain the therapeutic cornerstones for all arthritic conditions. Aspirin, or acetylsalicylic acid, belongs to a broad family of drugs known as salicylates that originates in plants like myrtle, willow, and coriander. Although ancient Egyptians and Assyrians used willow extract to reduce the redness and pain of inflamed joints, the first modern description of salicylate therapy didn't appear until several thousand years later. In 1763 Reverend Edward Stone of Oxfordshire, England, found that the pain and fever of malaria responded well to powdered willow bark suspended in water. The reverend had a curious rationale for using willow bark. He believed that God provided therapies for illnesses in the same environment where those illnesses abounded. Since both malaria and willow trees preferred moist climates, the willow must contain some cure for malaria.

A century after Stone's discovery, Thomas MacLagan of Dundee began treating "rheumatic miasma" with salicin acid, echoing Stone's reasoning. Moist climates—or so thought Dr. MacLagan—favored rheumatic illnesses (not technically true, but such climates do worsen the suffering of arthritics); plants from moist climates must therefore have the power to treat arthritis. Slurries of willow bark and other plant concoctions became the medical rage throughout Europe until a variety of wars and blockades made the supply of imported plant materials tenuous. As the demand for bark extracts grew, some enterprising chemists took it upon themselves to synthesize the active salicylates directly, bypassing the need for scarce plant resources.

Hermann Kolbe, a professor of chemistry at Marburg University, first succeeded in synthesizing salicylic acid, the precursor to modern aspirin, in industrial quantities in the late 1800s, selling it for one tenth the price of an equivalent amount of willow bark. Unfortunately, although salicylic acid could be applied externally, it proved too caustic for prolonged internal consumption, and the search for gentler salicylates continued.

In a strange twist of history, one patient disgusted with the indigestion caused by Kolbe's acid was entrepreneur Herr Hoffman, whose son worked as a chemist for a German manufacturer of chemical dyes, Fredrich Bayer & Company. The two Hoffmans synthesized a new drug, acetylsalicylic acid, that could be taken by mouth safely. The Bayer Company, although not strictly a pharmaceutical enterprise, instantly recognized the potential of the Hoffmans' new drug and on February 1, 1899, the company registered acetylsalicylic acid under the now-famous trade name Bayer Aspirin. The name Aspirin was a union of *a,* for "acetyl," and *spir,* for the plant "spirea ulmaria," the original source of salicylic acid.

Bayer immediately circulated information about its Aspirin to thousands of European physicians, launching the modern era of drug mass-marketing. Bayer also played hardball with competitors; if a physician wrote a prescription for Aspirin, the company demanded that only Aspirin be dispensed—other salicylate compounds could not be substituted. Originally dispensed as a powder, Aspirin became available in tablet form in 1904 and was soon on its way to being the most consumed drug on earth.

After World War I the victorious Allies sequestered Bayer's assets and promptly canceled Bayer's lucrative trademark protection on the name Aspirin. Bayer challenged this in the U.S. Supreme Court and lost, the Court deciding that Bayer was a victim of its own prosperity. Bayer had so effectively advertised its painkiller, the Court reasoned, that it no longer could claim proprietary ownership of the name. Aspirin with a small *a* passed into the realm of generic drugs in the United States and Great Britain, although Bayer maintains ownership of the name Aspirin in a number of other countries.

Today Americans consume forty *tons* of aspirin a day. It's used for everything from RA to migraines, from colds to postoperative pain. It also helps prevent strokes and heart attacks and may even reduce the incidence of Alzheimer's disease and colon cancer.

Aspirin is an anti-inflammatory drug. More specifically, it belongs to a family of anti-inflammatories known as nonsteroidals, or NSAIDs (nonsteroidal anti-inflammatory drugs). Spurred by the great success of aspirin, pharmacologists produced a menagerie of aspirin-like NSAIDs, including ibuprofen, indomethacin, naproxen, and many dozens more. Despite centuries of clinical use, no one knew how these drugs worked to reduced inflammation, until the early 1970s, when Vane and his coworkers showed that aspirin prevented the synthesis of a key inflammatory cytokine called prostaglandin E. Vane's discovery prompted researchers to look for other ways to block or neutralize the cytokines driving inflammation.

On the horizon today are two new classes of RA medications: COX-2 inhibitors, so named because they inhibit only the cyclooxygenase-2 enzyme, or COX-2, which generates prostaglandins; and Enbrel, a genetically engineered drug produced by Immunex Corporation of Seattle. Like aspirin, COX-2 inhibitors, called superaspirins, also block prostaglandin production (although they don't seem to have the same destructive effect on the stomach lining—their specificity for the COX-2 enzyme helps in this regard). Enbrel attacks another key cytokine: tumor necrosis factor (TNF). Despite its name, TNf plays an important role in "benign" diseases like RA.

→

For many patients, NSAIDs alone cannot control the pain and disability of RA; newer drugs like the superaspirins, although better than older compounds, will not cure the disease. When NSAIDs and gold therapy fail, arthritis experts turn to the most powerful (and most dangerous) weapons in their arsenal: steroids and immunosuppressives (chemotherapy drugs that cripple the immune system).

The body builds many different steroids from the same raw material, cholesterol, the dreaded artery clogger. For our purposes, steroids can be divided into two groups: corticosteroids and sex steroids. The body produces corticosteroids in the outer layer, or cortex, of the adrenal glands, the soft gray lumps sitting atop each kidney (the prefix *cortico-* is a variation of the word *cortex*). The testes and ovaries produce the bulk of our sex hormones. Corticosteroids protect us in times of stress, and sex steroids determine our secondary sexual characteristics, like beard growth in men. The widespread use of the nondescript word *steroids* can confuse patients taking the drugs. Women receiving corticosteroids for arthritic conditions, for example, may fear that they will grow large muscles and facial hair like female bodybuilders who use male sex steroids. In fact, corticosteroids actually cause muscle wasting, not muscle growth.

Corticosteroids are among the most powerful anti-inflammatory compounds known, making them indispensable tools in the treatment of autoimmune disorders. But like all potent drugs, they have a dark side, a side that remained hidden during the early days of steroid therapy. We have already seen in the stories of willow bark and gold therapy how wrongheaded theories of disease causation can still lead to useful remedies. Likewise, a mistaken theory of RA's origin resulted in the first use of corticosteroids in its treatment.

In the 1920s Dr. Philip Hench, a graduate of my alma mater, the University of Pittsburgh School of Medicine, observed that patients with underactive adrenal glands often had the same constitutional symptoms as RA patients. Hench concluded that RA was a form of adrenal hormone insufficiency and could be cured by hormone replacement. Diabetics lack insulin, so we give them insulin. RA patients lack corticosteroids, Hench argued, and so we need only give them corticosteroids and, voilà, a cure. In Hench's paradigm, steroid therapy would merely correct a natural deficiency in rheumatic patients, restoring them to normality; there would be no undesirable side effects.

Hench's theory couldn't be adequately tested until pure preparations of adrenal hormones became available. In the 1930s scientists extracted a pure hormone from human adrenal glands, calling it compound E. Given the limited supply of fresh human tissue, clinical use of compound E couldn't proceed until pharmacologists found a way of synthesizing it in the laboratory and preparing it in industrial quantities. After years of work, they finally achieved their goal, and by 1948 just enough compound E became available for Hench to perform a clinical trial in arthritis victims. His results were stunning. RA patients didn't just improve with compound E therapy—they became normal. Rheumatologists became convinced that Hench had been right all along. Compound E, renamed cortisone, was not just a treatment but a cure.

Hench and his coworker Kendall announced their bombshell findings in 1950 and, a scant one year later, received the Nobel Prize for their efforts, one of the quickest ever awarded (by comparison, Watson and Crick had to wait six years before getting their Nobel Prize for discovering the DNA double helix). The title of Hench's Nobel address, "The Reversibility of Certain Rheumatic and Non-rheumatic Conditions by the Use of Cortisone," shows that he, too, thought a cure had been found.

Note his bold use of the word *reversibility* instead of a more cautious term like *therapy*. The medical world shuddered with euphoria. RA had been conquered. Yet here sat my poor Clara, locked in a wheelchair and oblivious to the fact that Dr. Hench had apparently cured her disease over five decades earlier. What happened? Did his cure simply vanish?

Further trials proved that Hench had discovered only a short-term cure. The optimism of the early 1950s soon gave way to the realization that cortisone was far too malignant a drug for prolonged use. It worked miracles temporarily—there wasn't any doubt about that—but the long-term complications proved disastrous. His RA sufferers had entered into a Faustian contract with cortisone: it made them feel better now but caused awful consequences later on. Neither the Nobel committee nor the medical community at large had waited long enough before jumping on Hench's bandwagon.

Hench's original thesis—a deficiency of naturally produced cortisone causes RA—failed the test of time. In reality, RA patients make their own cortisone in sufficient amounts; contrary to Hench's theory, they have no hormonal deficiencies. To see any improvement in their arthritis, they must therefore consume an excess of cortisone, an overdose in fact. Sustained over many months, this overdose produces muscle wasting, ulcer disease, obesity, cataracts, osteoporosis, hip fractures, increased susceptibility to infections, poor healing of wounds, diabetes, and major personality changes. Since RA rarely causes death, patients must live with their disease for decades, and a safe arthritis medication must be tolerated for a lifetime, not just for a few blissful months.

So why use steroids at all? Because in advanced RA, the health risks of the disease itself often outweigh the risk of corticosteroids. Clara had been on the synthetic steroid prednisone in low doses for three years, with good results and tolerable side effects—Hench's Nobel Prize wasn't completely unwarranted. Early rheumatologists erred in using high doses because, like Hench, they thought the disease could be cured and therefore pushed the doses higher and higher until the patient was free of all symptoms. Modern rheumatologists use steroids more judiciously, searching for that dose providing the most improvement and the least side effects.

Nevertheless, rheumatologists still hesitate to use corticosteroids in the average RA patient. There is, after all, an ethical concern about giving patients a drug that makes them feel very good for a brief time, only to rescind it later when side effects flare up. I vaguely remember an old television show (a *Twilight Zone* episode perhaps) in which a man, blind from birth, must decide whether to undergo an operation that will allow him to see—but only for a day. Maybe, he reasons, it would be better never to see at all. The same dilemma faces the arthritis victim: how worthwhile is it to feel cured for a few months, then go back to the same old disease?

Once steroid therapy begins, the temptation to continue it forever in ever-increasing doses can be strong. Patients develop a kind of addiction to steroids, escalating their own doses without permission. Many of my brain tumor patients must take high doses of steroids just to survive, and I have personally witnessed the awful mayhem that these chemicals can inflict upon the human body. Strange as it may sound, the ravages of RA can appear mild compared to the ravages of steroids used to excess.

And so by the late 1950s, rheumatologists realized that cortisone, although a useful tool, wasn't the answer they had hoped it would be. Hollywood dramatized the dark underbelly of cortisone therapy in a 1956 film, *Bigger than Life*, starring James Mason.

Mason portrays a meek teacher diagnosed with polyarteritis no-
dosa, a lethal autoimmune disorder that attacks the arteries
within muscles and intestines. His doctors, flush with Henchian
enthusiasm, offer him experimental cortisone therapy, and Mason enjoys such immediate relief from his crippling bouts of
abdominal pain that he returns to his normal life and considers
himself cured. Unfortunately, the rising doses of corticosteroids
make him progressively more irritable and irrational. Doctors reduce the dosage, so he begins obtaining the medication under
false pretenses. The mild-mannered professor soon descends into
total madness and ends up attacking his own wife and family. In
the end he abandons cortisone therapy, preferring death as the
man he once was over life as the monster he had become. (High-
dose steroid therapy can indeed cause a "steroid psychosis" similar to that depicted in the film.)

There's an even more sinister side to the steroid story: Corticosteroids have been misused to exploit desperate RA victims.
Because the relief provided by steroids is so immediate and complete, while their troublesome side effects don't show up for several months or longer, they can be secretly made into bogus RA
cures. Patients pay big money for supposedly safe and natural
"home remedies" and see instant results; but by the time the char-
acteristic side effects of steroid overuse appear, the scam's perpe-
trators have closed up shop and moved on. For example, years ago
an unscrupulous Mexican RA clinic claimed to cure patients
with herbal preparations. The herbs worked so well that patients
flocked south of the border with money in hand to buy the
magical remedy. After taking the "herbs" for a few months
with remarkable results, a few patients began suffering mental
breakdowns similar to the one depicted in *Bigger than Life*—

subsequent chemical analysis of the magical herbs proved that they were nothing but cleverly disguised corticosteroid preparations.

➤

The biggest guns in the RA armamentarium are the immunosuppressives, drugs that weaken the body's defenses. These are the same agents used by transplant surgeons to prevent organ rejection. By crippling the immune system, physicians try to soften the blows RA rains upon the joints.

It's a dangerous gambit. Only the immune system stands between us and a world teeming with deadly microbes that would have us for lunch if given half a chance. Weakening the immune system to treat horror autotoxicus is like dismissing the police force to get rid of police brutality. It's an effective but risky strategy. Physicians must tread a fine line between not weakening the immune system enough, thereby leaving the disease untreated, and crippling it too much and exposing the patient to lethal infections.

To treat RA, rheumatologists commonly use methotrexate, a chemotherapy drug first introduced in the 1940s as a leukemia treatment. Therapies for RA and leukemia share a common goal—wiping out harmful white blood cells—and methotrexate plays a role in both diseases. The drug acts by interfering with folic acid; white cells exposed to the drug die of vitamin deficiency. A variety of other agents have been used to treat autoimmune diseases, including potent transplant drugs like azathioprine and cyclosporine.

Unfortunately, drugs like methotrexate rely on a "throw the

baby out with the bathwater" approach: they kill both good and bad white blood cells indiscriminately. The optimal RA therapy would target only the confused white cells responsible for attacking the victim's own synovium while leaving other cells unscathed. Such precision may be hard to achieve with drugs alone. Cypress Bioscience of San Diego has developed a more sophisticated approach: blood filtration. Using a device similar to a kidney dialysis machine, technicians remove blood from the patient's body, strip it of autoimmune white cells, and then return it. This elegant concept looks quite promising in early trials, but how long the effect lasts and whether it will warrant the price ($25,000 per treatment and up) remain open questions.

An article in the September 28, 1998, issue of *Time* magazine, "Arthritis Under Arrest," hailed new therapies like Enbrel, superaspirins, and blood filtration as "new therapies [that] may finally succeed in putting one of the worst forms of this painful illness on ice." I sincerely hope so, but we know from the unfortunate Hench affair that optimism can be premature. Let's hope history doesn't repeat itself.

Clara smiled and nodded patiently as I outlined the risks of my planned operation. Without the operation, I told her, her dying spine joints would continue to slide forward and soon her neck would snap under the weight of her own head. Clara was hanging herself using RA's rope, the ultimate horror autotoxicus, and I hoped to prevent this. But when I started to get into specific risks—infection, hemorrhage, paralysis—Clara raised her bent hand and stopped me.

"You've already told me that without this operation I will die. What more do I need to know?"

I explained that surgeons had to tell their patients all of the pertinent risks of surgery, even in those operations essential for saving their lives. She asked why; this seemed silly to her. "Because," I replied, "the courts of this country have decided that certain risks may be worse than death in the minds of some patients." For example, a person might prefer death over quadriplegia, a risk of the procedure I wanted to perform upon her. In our present "right to die" climate, we can't assume that a patient will choose an operation even in life-threatening situations. But she would have none of this.

"Some people only want to live if they're perfect. Well, I've learned that you can still do a lot of living even if you are far from perfect. If surviving means I have to have surgery, so be it."

Her surgery went smoothly. My orthopedic colleague and I lassoed her wandering Atlas to the vertebra below with two thick braids of metal wire, then tossed in bone chips harvested from her hip for good measure. Hopefully, the whole upper neck would meld into a safely immobilized mass of bone. At the conclusion of the procedure, we fitted her for a bulky brace and took her to the intensive care unit, where, unfortunately, her postoperative course was anything but smooth. Years of steroids had sapped her ability to heal. She developed a wound infection, then pneumonia. Her osteoporotic bone was slow to fuse. After she left the intensive care unit, the heavy neck brace made it difficult for her to walk on her steroid-weakened legs.

We decreased the steroid dose to hasten her wound healing, but the arthritis flared with a vengeance again. We doubled her aspirin dose, but this gave her a bleeding ulcer and she almost hemorrhaged to death. How difficult to fix a body bent on destroying itself from the inside out. We finally entered her in a rehabilitation center, where she would spend the next three months.

The fusion finally succeeded and she returned home. Clara did well for a number of years before yielding unexpectedly to a fulminant bladder infection. Her delinquent immune system failed her for the last time, letting in the invaders and permitting them to run wild.

She rests easily now, having fought the good fight. For almost half a century her body had been the battleground for a feud as old as life itself—the war between us and them; her addled immune system tilted like Don Quixote against the windmills of her crippled joints and then, at the very last, abdicated its responsibility and opened the drawbridge for the microbial barbarians waiting outside.

As she lay dying, her blood blazing with unchecked infection, I have no doubt that somewhere deep within her ravaged body her immune system finally understood how badly it had been duped all those miserable years.

"The horror," it cried, "the horror of it all."

7   THE STIGMATA

They have pierced my hands and my feet...

—Psalms 22:16

Lou was a milkman. He'd been delivering milk to private homes and local stores for over forty years, driving his first truck when milk came in bottles topped with cream and crimped foil. Back then nobody cared whether it was 1 percent or 2 percent fat; it was just plain milk. He was proud of his work—so few dairies provided home service nowadays—but much to his dismay, Lou hadn't been doing his job very well lately. Despite his die-hard work ethic, Lou had to call in sick at least once a week because of the gnawing pains in his wrists, arms, and shoulders. He feared he might lose his job, just two years shy of his planned retirement. He could fake some work injury, as his friends suggested, and ride out his remaining time on workers' compensation benefits. But he couldn't remember any injuries and he refused to lie about his condition. That just wasn't his nature. Besides, Lou couldn't see ending his long years as a working stiff that way, a disabled old man sitting at home collecting insurance money.

It all started with a vague aching in his wrists. He dismissed his aches as simple arthritis—until his fingers began to buzz. The pesky digits weren't quite asleep nor were they quite awake, and not all fingers were equally affected. His thumbs and the middle fingers—the ones Lou called his obscenity fingers—tormented him the most. Perhaps, he mused, the good Lord was punishing him for a lifetime of ill-tempered hand gestures.

The sensations didn't come all the time, only at night and when he drove his milk route. For months he awakened almost nightly with a searing numbness in both hands that wouldn't relent until he rose and paced the floor for an hour, clenching and unclenching his barking fingers as he walked. Sometimes that didn't work and he had to put his hands in the freezer until the numbness abated, often dozing off on a kitchen chair with his pajamas slick with melting ice. No one likes to lose sleep, least of all a man who had to be at work by five o'clock every morning, but Lou could deal with exhaustion. Driving his delivery truck—that was a different matter.

He found that he couldn't grasp the wheel for longer than five or ten minutes at a time. If he gripped it for any longer, his fingers would buzz and send pains rocketing up his arms into his shoulders. He would then be forced to release the wheel with the right hand and grip it with the left, then release it with the left and grip it with the right, back and forth, back and forth, in a painful dance that lasted for six solid hours as he made his required deliveries.

As the months wore on, the pains in his wrists, shoulders, and neck became more severe but the finger buzzing faded somewhat. As the buzzing lessened, he noticed that the hands didn't work as they should. He had trouble picking up coins and holding a coffee cup. Pencils would fly from his fingers as if possessed by demons. The wrists felt tight, like he was wearing handcuffs all the time, and his shoulder blades ached mercilessly.

A wounded Korean War veteran who prided himself on stoicism, Lou didn't relate these symptoms to his internist until he feared for his job. The internist, alarmed by the arm symptoms and how they worsened with activity, put Lou through an extensive cardiac evaluation and found nothing abnormal. This eased Lou's mind—he feared all along that his symptoms might be coming from his heart—but his infirmity remained undiagnosed.

Next stop: the orthopedic surgeon. By this time Lou's shoulder pain was more troublesome than his hand symptoms; the orthopedist diagnosed injuries to his rotator cuffs, the muscles that bind our arms to our shoulders. The cuffs become worn and frayed through overuse, leading to a grating mechanical pain. Although MRI scans of Lou's shoulders turned up little evidence of injury, the orthopedist remained unconvinced. She performed arthroscopy on his right shoulder, the worst one, by inserting a telescopic viewing device in the joint and examining the shoulder mechanism under direct vision. No pathology lurked there.

Next came an MRI of the neck, then a few steroid injections into the muscles of his shoulders followed by two six-week courses of physical therapy, all to no avail. Lou tried a home traction unit for his neck, heating pads, ginseng tea, chiropractic, even an acupuncture clinic advertised in his local newspaper, and still his arms and hands grew worse. Finally, his internist ordered a nerve conduction study of the arms, a sophisticated electrical analysis of nerve function, and discovered the source of his problem at last. It resided where the pain first began: in Lou's wrists.

Lou had that modern stigmata known as carpal tunnel syndrome, or CTS.

Stigmata comes from the Greek word meaning "to pierce or prick with a sharp object." In the Roman Catholic Church, *stigmata* refers to the six wounds of the crucified Jesus (nail wounds to the hands and feet, the thorn wounds of the scalp, and a postmortem lance wound to the right chest). People throughout history have claimed to be "stricken" with the stigmata, or at least with the nail wounds of the hands and feet. Those few who have been miraculously "stigmatized" became living saints, touring the countryside and allowing believers to touch their wounds. The first person to manifest the stigmata was Saint Francis of Assisi; in modern times, the most famous example was the Italian monk Padre Pio, who developed his stigmata in the early part of this century.

In a medical sense, CTS is a nonpenetrating version of the stigmata. I know comparing an orthopedic affliction to the wounds of Christ sounds strange, maybe even blasphemous to some, but it makes sense in the context of what we now know about ancient crucifixion. In most artistic depictions of the crucifixion, the nails have been driven through Christ's palms. Experiments with cadavers have shown, however, that a man crucified in this manner couldn't hang from a cross without the nails tearing out between the middle and ring fingers. There's insufficient strength in the skin and tissues of the palms to support an average man's weight. Moreover, the palms contain little nervous tissue. Nails driven there, assuming they missed the metacarpal bones, would be relatively painless, and painlessness isn't exactly what Christ's executioners had in mind.

As historian Jim Bishop argues in his book *The Day Christ Died,* Christ's executioners didn't drive the nails through his palms but through the wrists at the base of the thumb, in an area we now call the carpal tunnel (from the Latin *carpus,* meaning "wrist"). The heaviest body can hang indefinitely from nails driven through this area, thanks to the great strength of the ligaments binding the carpal bones together. Moreover, wrist nails lacerate the thick median nerve, so named because it courses down the middle of the arm like a highway's median strip. The pain generated by skewering these huge nerves with iron spikes must have defied description. (Incidentally, the Shroud of Turin, the controversial burial cloth allegedly imprinted with an image of the dead Christ, shows blood staining at the wrists, not the palms. Shroud devotees point to this as proof of its authenticity—medieval forgers should have depicted palmar, not carpal, nail wounds.) CTS acts like the nails of ancient executioners, crushing the median nerves at the wrists and producing incapacitating pain, numbness, and weakness in the hands, arms, shoulders, and neck.

Structurally, the carpal tunnel resembles an archer's bow. The small bones of the wrist form a flexible arch equivalent to the bow itself; stretched across this skeletal bow—the bowstring—is the transverse carpal ligament, a half-inch-thick band lying just beneath the skin at the base of the thumb. Ten cables pass through the channel formed by the wrist bones and carpal ligament: the median nerve and nine flexor tendons (two to each finger and one to the thumb). The tendons flex, or bend, the digits. The thumb gets only one flexing tendon because it has only one bendable joint compared to the fingers' two. Clench your fist very hard and observe the flexor tendons standing out beneath the thin skin of the wrist.

The median nerve is large, nearly the diameter of the smallest finger. Although we commonly think of nerves as wispy things, like fine wires or soft spaghetti strands, that isn't the case for the human median nerve. Thus, even inside a normal wrist, the carpal tunnel is a crowded place. As we age, our flexing tendons slowly thicken from repeated use, further crowding out the adjacent nerves. The transverse carpal ligament also enlarges with age, narrowing the diameter of the tunnel further. Eventually there's no room left for the nerve, and it becomes pinched by a vise of aging bone, ligament, and tendon. The nerve complains, sending electrical buzzing sensations into the thumb, index, and middle fingers (the ring and small finger tend to be less affected), and pain shooting retrograde into the shoulders, neck, upper back, and head. In advanced cases the nerve dies off, leaving behind a numb hand and a withered, useless thumb.

Like spinal disc disorders and childbirth pain, CTS is a uniquely human affliction, a by-product of our large opposable thumbs. All primates have opposing thumbs, of course, but the human thumb is unique even among higher apes. Compare a human hand to a chimpanzee's and note the striking differences in the thumb musculature. The base of the human thumb ripples with thick muscle while the chimp thumb appears flat and scrawny by comparison. (People with end-stage CTS are said to have a simian hand because of their atrophic thumb muscles.) Our overdeveloped thumb muscles give us greater pincer strength and finer hand control. The thumb's dominance can also be seen in the brain, where a disproportionate amount of cortical gray matter has been dedicated to the processing of thumb sensation and motion. Aside from the lower face and mouth, the thumb, index, and middle fingers are the most exquisitely sensitive structures in the entire body.

The median nerve serves as the brain's conduit to these sensitive areas, which explains its large dimensions. The nerve conveys the massive number of nerve fibers needed to control the magnificent mechanism formed by our thumbs and first two fingers. The ring and small fingers play only a minor role in hand dexterity and fall under the control of the smaller ulnar nerve, which lies outside the carpal tunnel. To see how unimportant the ring and small fingers are for dexterity, try knitting, buttoning a shirt, writing, or picking up a coin and note how these last two fingers tend to stay flexed and out of the way. All five digits contribute to gross grip strength, but our uniquely human dexterity resides largely in our thumbs, index, and middle fingers, and that's where CTS strikes hardest.

Unfortunately, our human need for mammoth median nerves also makes Homo sapiens prone to carpal tunnel compression syndromes. The large number of nerve cells dedicated to hand sensation also makes us hypersensitive to hand pain in the same way that a heavy nerve supply to the face and head makes us susceptible to headaches and facial tics. I believe CTS to be a direct consequence of our agile hands. The syndrome thus represents another human affliction arising from our unique anatomy. Childbirth pain stems from our big heads, disc disease from our upright posture, and CTS from our muscle-bound thumbs.

Philosophically, I find it intriguing that Jesus, who according to Christian teachings, came to earth to suffer human pain, died hanging by his two median nerves. The nails in his feet, the thorns in his head, even the scourging of his back would have produced pedestrian sufferings compared to that generated by his penetrating wrist wounds. Only in Homo sapiens could such small forelimb injuries prove so supremely punishing. Had Christ been stoned, drowned, or burned at the stake, his torment would have been no greater than any other animal enduring a similar fate. But crucifixion exploits a unique quirk of human anatomy: the funneling of a massive number of nerve fibers through a tiny wrist. Was humanity redeemed by CTS times two? A weird thought to be sure, but two thousand years later, Lou the milkman felt the spikes in his own wrists. Fortunately, medical science has discovered a simple way of prying them back out.

➤

Occupational physicians consider CTS a repetitive trauma syndrome often caused by work activities. According to this theory, excessive use of the fingers—as needed in occupations like typing, mail sorting, computer programming, assembly line work, and switchboard operation—causes repetitive microtrauma to the hands, predisposing workers to thickening of their finger tendons and greatly increasing their risk of disabling CTS. In the United States, CTS has become one of the most common "work-related" health problems, on a par with back injuries. Although work habits can certainly aggravate CTS and might possibly initiate it in some people, I disagree with the popular notion that occupational repetitive trauma *causes* the vast majority of CTS in industrialized nations. To be sure, working can be a miserable experience for people afflicted with CTS (as Lou discovered), but there are several reasons for rejecting the theory that the workplace spawns most CTS.

First, nearly all occupations require frequent use of the hands (with the possible exception of professional soccer), and yet not all professions are equally affected. Why are typists more prone to CTS than violinists or surgeons, professions that also require continuous finger activity?

Second, in my experience, CTS affects the nondominant

hand nearly as frequently as the dominant hand, which makes no sense in any repetitive trauma model of CTS. Lou, for example, had severe CTS in both hands simultaneously (which is surprisingly common). If excessive use of the hands was a major factor in CTS, the disease should overwhelmingly favor the right hand, given the large proportion of right-handed people, and it doesn't. Although overuse does contribute to arthritic syndromes in joints, the mechanical demands placed on finger tendons can't compare to the strains suffered by weight-bearing structures.

Third, CTS occurs two to three times more commonly in women, particularly middle-aged women; I find it unlikely that the fondness of CTS for middle-aged females stems from sex differences in the workplace, although occupational factors can't be completely ruled out. Even in this enlightened age, women still dominate allegedly "at-risk" groups such as typists and computer keyboard operators. Nevertheless, the smaller diameter of the female wrist, together with the higher incidence of rheumatic diseases in women, may have more to do with a woman's risk of CTS than disparities in occupation.

Fourth, the incidence of CTS varies according to the willingness of insurance companies and governments to recognize it as a compensable work injury. A major "outbreak" of a CTS-like pain syndrome occurred in Australia in the 1980s after the government recognized repetitive trauma as a disability worthy of government subsidy. The outbreak faded soon after coverage for repetitive trauma injuries became harder to obtain. As in other work injuries, insurance fraud and malingering have made it difficult to tell whether CTS is a legitimate occupational injury or simply a ubiquitous degenerative process exploited by disgruntled workers for monetary gain. Lou's CTS made his job more difficult, but he refused to claim that his job gave him a disease. Other patients may not be so honest, especially when faced with termination and loss of income.

Finally, CTS becomes most symptomatic during periods of hand rest, not periods of hand overactivity. Again, this is at odds with the repetitive trauma model. CTS usually strikes at night when the hands are immobile, often waking patients out of a deep sleep. As Lou discovered, driving is also a problem since it requires the hands to be held motionless on a steering wheel for long periods of time. The symptoms can be relieved by repeatedly opening and closing the hand, the same maneuvers that occupational experts claim cause the disease in the first place.

There's a simple explanation for the worsening of CTS with hand inactivity. We rely on the constant motion of our fingers to squeeze blood out of the hands and back to the heart. Even ten or fifteen minutes of finger immobility produces blood pooling in the wrists and hands, causing them to swell imperceptibly. Or perceptibly in some cases; go on a bike ride and feel how stiff and swollen your fingers can become after being held motionless below the level of your heart. This swelling "tips the scales" in patients with tight carpal tunnels, worsening their symptoms. The tendency of women to retain water in synchrony with the menstrual cycle may be an additional reason why they are more prone to CTS than men.

To reverse the swelling, patients pump excess blood from their carpal tunnels by clenching and unclenching their hands repeatedly, literally wringing excess fluids out of the tissues. If that fails, the hands can be iced down like a sprained ankle. One of my patients could get relief only by kneading raw ground beef. He kept a pound of the stuff in his refrigerator at all times just for that purpose.

He ate a lot of meat loaf and burgers before he finally agreed to surgery.

⤜

Whatever its cause, CTS is fairly easy to treat in most cases. Although it now ranks as the number one problem affecting the hand, surgeons only recognized it as a defined syndrome in the 1940s and didn't even coin the phrase *carpal tunnel syndrome* until the 1950s.

The earliest descriptions of anything sounding like CTS appeared in the late 1800s. At that time physicians referred to CTS as acroparesthesia of the hand, but no one had a clue what caused it until 1913, when French physicians Marie and Foix observed that the median nerves in a few cadavers seemed squashed in the carpal tunnel. They proposed that mechanical compression of the median nerve could be a surgically correctable cause of acroparesthesia and astutely suggested cutting the transverse carpal ligament in patients with median nerve dysfunction in the hand. Unfortunately, the medical community promptly ignored their stunningly prophetic proposal.

The first surgical treatments for CTS didn't take place until the 1920s, almost two decades after Marie and Foix's work. Early surgeons misunderstood the anatomy of the carpal tunnel and often damaged key branches of the nerve during surgery. Their poor results discouraged widespread surgical therapy of CTS for many years. In fact, safe surgery for CTS didn't become widely available until after 1960, when pioneers like Mayo Clinic orthopedist George Phalen (who, incidentally, coined the phrase *carpal tunnel syndrome*), refined the modern carpal tunnel release. This simple procedure evolved into one of the most successful operations done for any disease on any part of the body. Like spinal disc surgery, carpal tunnel surgery has an astounding benefit-to-risk ratio when appropriately applied and ranks among the least-heralded wonders of the surgical world.

As Marie and Foix theorized nearly a century ago, CTS can be cured simply by surgically dividing the transverse carpal ligament. This maneuver permits the wrist bones to spring open slightly like a bow straightening after the bowstring is cut, thereby affording the contents of the carpal tunnel a few precious millimeters of additional breathing space. In greater than 90 percent of patients, these extra few millimeters relieve all CTS symptoms within days or weeks of surgery, so long as the nerves haven't been irrevocably damaged by the CTS. Fortunately, such permanent nerve damage from CTS is rare.

Like any operation, carpal tunnel release has changed somewhat over the years. In the early 1960s surgeons opened the hand and not only cut the transverse ligament but also laboriously separated the nerve from the tendons to remove "scar tissue." This tedious dissection often lasted hours and required general anesthesia. Postoperatively, patients wore casts on their hands for weeks and then, after the casts were removed, needed many months of hand therapy to alleviate the postoperative stiffness in their fingers.

In the 1970s surgeons simplified the procedure somewhat. They confined themselves to cutting only the transverse ligament (what Marie and Foix first suggested), a task that could be completed under local anesthesia in fifteen or twenty minutes. Patients wore soft dressings for a few weeks and rarely needed any therapy. Final results were as good or better than those achieved with more radical surgery.

In the 1990s CTS surgery became even more minimalist. Surgeons now thread a tiny knife through a small nick in the skin and, with the aid of a tiny endoscope, cut the transverse ligament via remote control without the need for a large incision over the wrist and palm. Theoretically, patients treated with this minimalist approach can return to their regular activities within days. From a practical point of view, there is little evidence that the endoscopic approach affords any lasting advantage over the lower technology operation of the 1980s and the latter remains the most commonly used procedure today.

Surgery isn't the first option for CTS, of course. (Knife wounds to the heart aside, surgery is rarely the first option for any disease.) In mild cases it can be treated or even cured by a trial of wrist splinting. Flexing the hand at the wrist places strain on the median nerve and worsens the pain of CTS; wrist splints prevent this. One study also found that taking B vitamins may help early CTS, too, but this has not been confirmed by other investigators, and the theory that CTS results from vitamin deficiency remains controversial. Overdosing with B vitamins can actually cause further nerve damage and so this approach cannot be recommended.

If splints don't work, steroid injections into the carpal tunnel can be tried. These work, but only temporarily in my experience; they also carry some risk of nerve injury. For patients in whom splints fail or with signs of median nerve damage (permanent finger numbness, thumb wasting, clumsiness of the hand), surgery should be considered the next option. Although not without risk, surgery's hazards are so far outweighed by its benefits that the operation should not be delayed once the diagnosis is made and a brief trial of nonsurgical therapy tried.

Diagnosis of CTS should be straightforward. CTS produces such a stereotypical clinical picture that experienced hand surgeons can often diagnose it with confidence over the phone. On examination, the presence of thumb weakness, finger numbness, a positive Phalen's sign (increased pain and numbness with forced wrist flexion), or a positive Tinel's sign (tingling in the fingers produced by striking the wrist with a reflex hammer) seals the diagnosis. Measuring the electrical conductance of the median nerve (the nerve conduction test, or NCV, that finally diagnosed Lou) provides objective evidence of median nerve injury and can quantitate the severity of the carpal tunnel compression.

Lou's physicians didn't think of CTS when they first evaluated him, because they fell victim to the common misconception that CTS is a "trivial" disease incapable of causing so much misery. They searched for more "serious" causes of Lou's arm pain, including a ruptured disc in the neck, cardiac angina, and shoulder trauma. When I told Lou and his internist that I thought his headaches, neck pains, shoulder pains, arms pains, and hand numbness all originated in his wrists, both scoffed at me. But his final outcome proved them happily wrong.

Lou's NCV revealed that his nerves had already endured extensive damage, and I was forced to take him to surgery straightaway. I released both hands at two operations spaced three weeks apart. His shoulder pain ceased on the operating table as I sliced his transverse ligaments with a pointed scalpel. Through my telescopic lenses, I watched as his choked median nerves sprang forth from their prisons and pulsated with new life. Lou went back to work a month after his hands healed and delivered his milk free of discomfort for the remaining years leading up to his retirement.

＊

All peripheral nerves must pass through channels of ligament, muscle, and bone on their way to their final destinations. Consequently, any nerve in the body can become entombed in degenerating tissue, tumors, bone fractures, surgical scars, or some combination of these processes. We have already seen how an atherosclerotic artery can crush the trigeminal nerve and how spinal nerves may be distorted by displaced disc cartilage. In the extremities, nerves are most vulnerable at anatomic bottlenecks like the carpal tunnel. The resulting "entrapment neuropathies" can cause significant suffering in otherwise healthy people.

Carpal tunnel is by far the most common form of entrapment neuropathy, but there are many others. The second most common nerve entrapment in the arm involves the ulnar nerve at the inner aspect of the elbow (the "funny bone"). As mentioned previously, the ulnar nerve supplies the ring and small fingers. At the elbow, the nerve runs just beneath the skin, where it can be easily bruised. The intense pain caused by striking the funny bone comes from concussion of this poorly protected nerve. The nerve can also be damaged by rapidly rotating the wrist, which causes a bone in the elbow to strum the nerve like a guitar pick strumming a string. That's why forcibly twisting a doorknob or opening a recalcitrant jar lid can occasionally send shocks of pain from the elbow down to the little finger.

When we repeatedly rest our elbows on firm, flat surfaces, scar tissue forms that can compress the nerve. Our sedentary lifestyles put the ulnar nerves at risk. We stress the nerves for long periods by reading in bed with our elbows pressed against the bed surface or by driving long distances with our elbows propped on hard armrests. Over time, cumulative elbow trauma causes symptomatic entrapment. Surgical release of scar tissue encasing the nerve usually produces a cure, although ulnar nerve release doesn't have the same high success rate produced by CTS release at the wrist.

Like CTS, ulnar neuropathy at the elbow (also called cubital tunnel syndrome or—because of its prevalence in people who like to rest their elbows on bars—beer drinkers' palsy) can produce arm pain, shoulder pain, and headache. For patients wishing to avoid surgery, I advise wearing the bulky foam elbow pads used by football players, for several weeks. Simple lifestyle adjustments, like resting the arms on soft pillows when driving, can also fix an aching ulnar nerve.

Less common entrapments include tarsal tunnel syndrome (the equivalent of CTS in the foot), Guyon's entrapment (ulnar nerve compression at the wrist), Morton's neuroma (compression of a tiny nerve between two toes), and meralgia paresthetica, a painful numbness of the outer thigh resulting from compression of the lateral femoral cutaneous nerve in the outer groin. This last syndrome, which I myself suffer from occasionally, comes from tight belts and other constrictive clothing or, as in my case, from excessive abdominal fat folding over the inguinal area. The only meralgia patient I ever treated who had a washboard abdomen got the disease from a low-hanging toolbelt. After I advised him to hang his tools from suspenders instead of a belt, his meralgia disappeared. (Unfortunately, his shoulders began to hurt because of the suspenders. He just couldn't win.)

Meralgia paresthetica also occurs occasionally after hernia

surgery or after spinal fusions wherein a bone graft has been harvested from the anterior hip. In these instances, the cutaneous nerve becomes entrapped by an incisional scar. Like CTS, the clinical picture of meralgia looks the same in all patients, regardless of causation. Patients complain of dense (and I mean very dense) numbness of the thigh from the groin to the knee, sometimes accompanied by pain in the leg, hip, or back. The condition may be permanent or episodic, with periods of numbness triggered by body position. In my case, lying flat for more than ten or twenty minutes precipitates thigh numbness. Standing can also bring on the numbness in some patients.

In any entrapment neuropathy, local steroid injections or decompressive surgeries usually provide lasting relief so long as the diagnosis is made in a timely fashion. Unfortunately, many primary care physicians lack the experience and neurological background to recognize entrapment neuropathies. Most meralgia patients, for example, end up misdiagnosed as suffering lumbar disc herniations because their physicians have been misled by the large amount of pain and numbness in the legs. My meralgia patients often undergo extensive back therapy and lumbar nerve blocks before the proper diagnosis occurs. A great number of CTS patients put up with meaningless physical therapy and chiropractic manipulations of their necks before someone finally identifies the source of their complaints.

Given the large number of misdiagnosed CTS patients, it's easy to see how more obscure entrapments like meralgia and Guyon's palsy can go undiagnosed for months, even years. Truly rare conditions, like posterior interosseus nerve entrapment in the forearm, can puzzle even the most experienced experts.

Over the years I have learned that CTS and other nerve entrapments are far from trivial diseases. Those who bear the modern stigmata endure innumerable days spent in pain and nights spent without sleep. When these patients complain to their doctors, however, they face the same problem Jesus faced when meeting the doubting Thomas: disbelief. These wounds can't be real.

How can such normal, healthy-looking people have so many complaints, many doctors wonder. Hand numbness? Big deal. Well, it can be a very big deal indeed. The median nerves are life-lines to our hands, and our hands a link to the physical world. Numb hands are like blind eyes.

Fortunately, we need no miracles to make them see again.

8   ANCIENT PAINS

"They say the poor countess is very ill.
The doctor says it is angina pectoris."

"Angina? Oh, that's a terrible illness!"

—Leo Tolstoy, *War and Peace*

My father has suffered from intermittent left arm and chest pain for years. The pains began when he was forty-five years old; his physicians first diagnosed a herniated cervical disc and prescribed physical therapy and a home traction unit. I was in high school at the time, and I recall thinking how ridiculous he looked in that traction device, a Rube Goldberg contraption consisting of a bag of water slung over a metal pulley attached to the bathroom door. The weight of the water yanked on a collar slung under the head and chin, thereby stretching the neck and, according to accepted theory, taking the strain off a sagging neck disc. He thought the thing was ridiculous, too, and it certainly afforded him little relief.

The pains waxed and waned for nine years, always bothersome but never disabling. Just some "creepy" form of neuralgia, he would say (none of us knew what a neuralgia was, let alone a creepy neuralgia, and I'm sure he didn't, either). Then one morning as he rose to go to work, the pains came hard...harder than ever. He thought an elephant was sitting on his chest and he noted a vague choking sensation in his throat. He fought to catch his breath and went downstairs to get something to eat despite a touch of nausea. As he sat with his morning coffee, the pains intensified further and a sense of dread overwhelmed him. He knew this was no ordinary illness. This was something mortal; his life was in jeopardy. My mother took one look at his moist, ashen face and came to the same realization. My father, the man who virtually never missed work or admitted he was ill, quietly asked to be taken to the nearest hospital.

Regardless of their medical sophistication, most people will recognize what ailed my father on that bleak autumn morning. He suffered a heart attack, more correctly known as myocardial infarction, or MI. The pains that plagued him all those years didn't come from a bad cervical disc or from creepy neuralgia, but from angina, the heart's cries of impending disaster.

Angina signifies an inadequate blood supply to the beating heart and results from atherosclerotic clogging of the heart's coronary arteries, vessels that derive their name from the Latin word *corona,* meaning "crown." The arteries form a jagged crown encircling the top of the heart.

The pains of angina vary in character and magnitude from person to person. My father's version was fairly typical: a faint squeezing sensation in the center of the chest together with aching in the left arm and shoulder. Other areas commonly affected by anginal pains include the neck, the jaw, and the space between the shoulder blades. The pain distribution of angina varies somewhat depending upon which part of the heart has the poorest oxygen supply. Pain from the rear of the heart, for example, tends to radiate to the patient's back, while pain from the base of the heart—the area abutting the diaphragm—goes into the shoulders.

Oddly, some people feel no cardiac pain at all. My father's best friend died from cardiac disease, yet he never had an anginal episode in his life. Testing showed that he had suffered two or three major heart attacks late in life, but he couldn't remember any of them. Lifelong diabetics seem particularly vulnerable to this painless form of coronary disease. Conversely, some patients suffer awful bouts of angina even though their coronary arteries barely show any disease.

Medical science didn't acknowledge the heart's role in pumping blood until Harvey's landmark treatise on circulation appeared in 1628. Despite their ignorance of physiology, ancient healers began diagnosing and treating chest pain as early as the fifth century. Even in the Dark Ages, physicians recognized the common association of severe chest discomfort, anxiety, and shortness of breath; a few astute clinicians even ascribed these symptoms to the heart itself, although they could deduce little else given their limited knowledge.

The use of the word *angina* for recurrent bouts of coronary insufficiency started with renowned London internist William Heberden in 1768. In an address to the Royal College of Physicians, Heberden coined the phrase *angina pectoris,* which we now commonly shorten to *angina. Angina* was an ancient medical term even in Heberden's day. It comes from the nasalized Indo-European root *angh* meaning "to choke" or, alternately, "to suffer." In Latin, *angh* became *angina,* a word Roman healers used in its literal sense—choking—to describe inflammatory diseases of the throat. In modern English, *angh* spawned a menagerie of similar words, including *angst, anguish, anger, anxiety,* and *ache.* Heberden, like the Romans, used *angina* in its "choking" context; his phrase *angina pectoris* loosely translates as a choking in the chest.

Angh implies much more than the simple physical act of choking. The word also refers to the feelings of panic and doom that accompany strangulation and drowning, which explains the modern conversion of *angh* to emotional words like *anguish* and *anxiety.* Heberden's choice of *angina* couldn't have been more appropriate in this sense. He knew that cardiac pain had both a physical and an emotional side and that these two sides could not be easily separated. A patient suffering severe cardiac strangulation feels not only pain, but a morbid fear of imminent death as well.

The underlying cause of anginal pain is *ischemia,* a word formed by the Greek words *ischo* (to keep back) and *haima* (blood). Ischemia results when blood flow to a given body part fails to satisfy that part's requisite oxygen, glucose, and waste disposal needs. In economic terms, ischemia represents a gross imbalance of blood supply and nutrient demand. Usually this means inadequate supply—the reduction or cessation of blood flow—but ischemia can also result from excessive demand. Cramping in athletes, for example, is a form of muscle ischemia in which the demand for oxygen in overexercised limbs exceeds the ability of healthy arteries to provide it.

After being deprived of blood flow, all tissues fall back into a survivalist mode by reducing their metabolic rate, drawing on reserves of stored food, retaining wastes, and burning fuel anaerobically (without the need for oxygen). How long cells can survive this way depends upon the type of cell it is. Cells with very high metabolic needs, like nerve cells and working cardiac muscle cells, can survive for only a few minutes at best without an influx of fresh blood. Cells with lower metabolic demands—like skin cells, liver cells, and resting muscle cells—can last for an hour or longer without blood flow before dying. If they are cooled to slow their metabolic rates further, they might even last a day sans blood.

In peripheral nerves and muscle, including the nonskeletal muscles comprising the heart and intestinal walls, ischemia causes severe pain. Curiously, in nonmuscular internal organs like the brain, liver, and kidneys, ischemia occurs silently. Cardiac ischemia—angina—produces dreadful discomfort, while the largest brain stroke is an entirely painless affair. This organ-dependent variability in the sensation of ischemic pain turns out to be a very practical adaptation. Nature gives us ischemic pain only when we can do something constructive to reverse it.

The ischemic pain of marathon runners forces them to stop running and reduce their metabolic demands before irreversible muscle injury occurs. When we fall asleep on one of our arms in an awkward position and kink off its blood supply totally, the ensuing ischemic pain wakes us and forces us to move about. Ischemic pain in a man with coronary disease makes him cease shoveling snow, alleviating the strain on his overloaded ventricles. The blood supply and metabolic demands of the heart, muscles, and nerves fall under our control, at least to some degree, making ischemic pain a useful tool. I can decrease the blood flow to my buttocks by sitting on a hard surface for two hours—until they hurt and turn numb; I can then increase buttock blood supply by getting off my posterior again. Likewise, I can reduce the metabolic demand to my heart by resting and increase it by walking to the top of the Empire State Building. Ischemic pain provides necessary feedback to our conscious minds, alerting us to dangerous imbalances in metabolic supply and demand.

For most internal organs, however, we cannot alter blood flow or metabolic demand with conscious behavior; ischemic pain in these organs would serve no purpose other than to act as cruel and unnecessary punishment. For example, there's nothing we can do to limit a cerebral stroke in progress. The brain runs its engines at full throttle all the time, day and night, and will sputter to a standstill within minutes of running short of fuel. What good would stroke pain accomplish? We have been endowed with ten times more liver and kidney tissue than we need to survive, making liver and kidney "strokes" largely harmless. Painful warnings of liver and kidney strokes are likewise superfluous.

Ischemic pain molds our day-to-day existence by telling us how much we can exercise, how long we can sit in one position, and what postures are safe for sleeping. But in certain disease conditions, ischemic pain does more than alter our lives. It can rule them.

⟶

Angina remains, far and away, the most common disabling ischemic pain syndrome. Although all muscle tissue hurts when deprived of sufficient oxygen, cardiac muscle appears particularly sensitive to ischemic pain. When made ischemic (or dead) by poor coronary blood flow, even tiny bits of cardiac muscle scream out with a pain capable of knocking the strongest people to their knees. An equivalent amount of ischemic biceps muscle causes only nuisance pain by comparison.

And who ever heard of a "biceps attack" from ischemia in the first place? Why is the heart, the most precious pound of muscle in our bodies, so prone to ischemia and ischemic pain? The obvious answer: cardiac muscle contracts all the time, every minute of every day from birth until death, while the lowly biceps gets to take nice long siestas (unless its Arnold Schwarzenegger's biceps, which seem to work round the clock). But this answer is only partially correct; the complete answer gets a bit more complicated.

Cardiac muscle has less collateral blood supply than skeletal muscle. Collateralization refers to how many different avenues blood can take to reach a given organ. Skeletal muscles have excellent collateral blood supplies because they reside in moving parts—like arms and legs—and cannot depend on one or two arteries for their nutrition. Mechanical bending of a limb kinks off arteries; to insure a steady flow of blood during activity, skeletal muscles have been given a wealth of nutrient arteries. No matter what position the arm or leg takes, at least one artery remains open. Thus, heavy collateralization buffers skeletal muscles against the transient occlusions that occur during limb movement. The situation is analogous to traffic going in and out of a major city. Wise urban planners allow for collateral traffic routes so that traffic won't become hopelessly snarled if one or two roads close due to accidents or construction.

Enclosed by vaults of bone and relatively impervious to bodily motion, the heart and brain have surprisingly poor collateral blood supplies. If one cerebral or coronary artery occludes, the healthy arteries that remain cannot take up the slack and ischemia quickly ensues. This seems paradoxical, even absurd: the biceps is better equipped to deal with ischemia than the heart and brain? But remember, we weren't designed to live forever.

Because of the heart's lackluster collateral supply, even small degrees of coronary narrowing can cause clinical angina or even frank MI. Moreover, the sophisticated electrical architecture of the heart makes even the smallest cardiac injury life threatening. Although it looks more like a piece of strip steak than a computer, the heart possesses a brain of its own. The billions of individual muscle fibers must contract in a coordinated rhythm so that the chamber walls move as a single unit. If anything disturbs this delicate synchronicity, heart fibers start marching out of step with one another and the heart turns to a quivering mass incapable of propelling blood, a lethal state known as ventricular fibrillation.

Regions of ischemic heart muscle, regardless of their size, can generate aberrant electrical impulses capable of igniting fibrillation. This is yet another reason why the heart has a greater sensitivity to ischemia than the biceps muscle. Unlike the heart, the biceps has no cybernetic function; small injuries to limb muscles have no life-threatening sequelae. Minute heart injuries, on the other hand, can be exceedingly dangerous because they increase the risk of wholesale fibrillation. Even injuries too small to affect the heart's contractile strength can result in electrical gridlock and death.

Consequently, our bodies will not tolerate any degree of cardiac ischemia, no matter how seemingly trivial. At the first signs of coronary insufficiency, the heart begins pestering its owner to make lifestyle changes. The sensitive nature of heart muscle and the ubiquitous nature of coronary atherosclerosis combine to make angina a daily burden for millions of people.

Angina worsens during activities that increase the heart's workload. The pain escalates until the angina victim can't continue doing stressful activities anymore—precisely the outcome the heart seeks. By reducing the rate and force of contraction, pain-enforced cardiac rest reduces the degree of ischemia and lowers the risk of fatal electrical miscues. Unfortunately, the angina victim and his heart aren't always "on the same page" in this regard. The heart wants to rest; the patient wants to get going. The patient wants to have sexual intercourse and play tennis, while the heart prefers avoidance of these activities. The patient wants to watch a Steelers game, but the heart knows that the large blood pressure surges that occur during inopportune fumbles and interceptions may lethally burden its poorly oxygenated left ventricle (I've had the dubious honor of watching a patient go into a fumble-induced ventricular fibrillation during a play-off game).

The desire to do more than the heart allows sends the typical sufferer to the doctor. For hundreds of years, though, this did little more than enrich doctors. The only treatment for angina was rest and more rest, together with large doses of narcotics or sedatives for extreme cases. Medieval doctors also employed leeching and bleeding, which worked surprisingly well in some cases (probably by lowering blood pressure). None of these constitutes palatable therapy for the modern patient-on-the-go.

The first real breakthrough in anginal pain therapy occurred in 1857, when Dr. T. Lauder Brunton discovered that inhalation of amyl nitrate completely relieved severe angina for up to a minute. Try as he could, though, Brunton could not find a way to extend this relief beyond sixty blissful seconds. Because of its brief duration and unpredictable dosing, amyl nitrate proved a very impractical cardiac drug. Twenty years later William Murrell, searching for a longer-acting version of amyl nitrate, experimented with a stable form of the explosive nitroglycerin. Nitroglycerin proved so successful in ameliorating angina that Murrell advocated taking the drug prophylactically. Heart patients could now take a pill before physical activity and proceed without fear of pain. The medical world was astounded.

Over a century has passed since Murrell's discovery, and angina patients the world over still carry the trusty nitroglycerin tablets in their pockets. In fact, the 1998 Nobel Prize went to three scientists who discovered, among other things, how nitroglycerin works. The drug is a vasodilator—it causes arteries to expand in diameter. Nitroglycerin provokes dilation by stimulating the production of a natural substance, nitrous oxide (yes, laughing gas), within the cells lining the arteries. Nitrous oxide induces relaxation in muscular arterial walls and increases the size of the artery, augmenting blood flow. Nitrous oxide plays a critical role in many vascular diseases, including coronary disease, brain hemorrhages, and impotence. (The anti-impotence drug Viagra also acts via nitrous oxide, thereby increasing blood flow to the penis and facilitating erection.)

Nitroglycerin does *not* dilate coronary arteries, however, and has no direct effect on blood flow to the heart. So how does it relieve angina? Amazingly enough, by dilating arteries everywhere else. By opening all of the arteries in the body at once, nitroglycerin reduces the amount of oxygen-consuming work the beating heart must do. Try exhaling through a garden hose, then try exhaling through a drinking straw. Notice how much easier it is to blow through a large bore tube compared to a small bore tube. Likewise, the heart can more easily drive blood through dilated arteries than constricted arteries. Nitroglycerin reduces the amount of oxygen the heart needs to pump the same amount of blood, balancing supply-and-demand imbalance by reducing demand, not by increasing supply. Regrettably, the global arterial dilation produced by nitroglycerin does have a bad side effect: throbbing headaches.

Despite the bad headaches, nitroglycerin ranks alongside aspirin as one of the true miracle drugs of our age. Prior to the advent of other antianginal drugs in the middle of this century and the perfection of coronary bypass in the 1960s, nitroglycerin was the mainstay of heart therapy. As we honor today's physicians for their work on AIDS and cancer drugs, let's not forget pioneers like Murrell. To put Murrell's discovery in perspective: for modern physicians to lay claim to an achievement as great as Murrell's, millions of patients must be using the drugs they discover today in the year 2120. Feats like the discovery of aspirin and nitroglycerin are not likely to be repeated in our lifetimes.

Although less prone than cardiac muscle to ischemia, skeletal muscle will also cause ischemic pain when deprived of circulation. Hardening of the leg arteries with age results in a progressive inability to walk due to severe pain and cramping in the calves, a condition known as claudication, from the Latin *claudicatio*, meaning "to limp." (Fans of the Robert Graves novel and PBS series of the same name, *I, Claudius*, will remember the limping gait of Roman Emperor Claudius I.)

The first steps in treating both vascular claudication and angina involve lifestyle changes: reduction of fat intake, cessation of smoking, and better control of hypertension through medications and the regulation of salt intake. A progressive exercise program may help both heart and leg muscles to increase their collateral blood supply. Thinning agents like aspirin or warfarin can prevent sludging of blood in narrowed arteries and reduce ischemia. If these nonsurgical methods fail, surgical opening or bypassing of clogged arteries can be tried.

↠

We took my father to our local hospital. Luckily, his heart attack proved to be quite small; nevertheless, his cardiologist transferred him to a major medical center, where he underwent urgent bypass surgery. Several years later he suffered a second attack—one of the vein grafts occluded—and needed a second bypass operation. At the second procedure, surgeons took the mammary arteries supplying his inner chest wall and redirected them into his left anterior descending coronary artery. (Because skeletal tissues have so many collateral sources of blood, stealing a major artery like the mammary and plugging it into the heart will not harm the chest muscles.) Now, eight years after this last procedure, he remains pain free in his retirement and can walk an eighteen-hole golf course daily. He still keeps a bottle of nitroglycerin handy, just in case. Dr. Murrell still lives in his golf bag.

⤛

Nineteenth-century neurologist Sir Henry Head had a lifelong fascination with the human sensory system. A fanatic about studying sensation, Head actually cut one of the major sensory nerves in his own left arm in order to study the numbness left behind. They don't make researchers like Sir Henry anymore. Head, among others, pioneered the concept that sensation is not one entity but many different entities, each with its own unique dimension: pain, touch, vibratory sense, temperature sense.

Head further subdivided pain sensation into two subtypes: epicritic and protopathic. Epicritic pain (from the Greek, *epikritikos*, meaning "to judge") is sharp and easily localized to a specific region of the body; protopathic pain (from the Greek *proto*, "first," and *pathos*, "suffering") is dull and poorly localized. I currently have a paper cut at the very tip of my left middle finger. I can

close my eyes and tell within a millimeter exactly where it is—
that's epicritic pain.

Angina and other so-called "visceral" pains are protopathic.
Protopathic pains tend to spread out over large areas of the body.
Patients state "my belly hurts" or "my chest hurts" and can't localize their discomfort any further. Anatomically, the pathways
that carry epicritic pain evolved only recently. Conversely, the
pathways conveying protopathic pain are among the oldest in the
nervous system (hence the name, "first suffering"). Protopathic
pains are ancient pains, pains dating back eons in time.

Epicritic pains—lacerations, ankle sprains, fractures—come
from external traumas, while protopathic pains—angina, gallbladder attacks, kidney stones, stomach ulcers—have their origins in internal disease and dysfunction. Protopathic pains are the
body's megaphone, a way of telling the brain that something's
gone bad within the inner clockwork. The brain's need-to-know
regarding malfunctions of the body must have evolved in parallel
with the brain itself, that's why protopathic pains travel through
such ancient circuitry. Protopathic pains were the first pains and,
for a time, the only pains.

The ancient pain pathways used by protopathic sensations
intertwine with the equally primitive pathways regulating the
autonomic functions of the body: sweating, gastric and intestinal
motility, heart rate, respiratory rate, and vascular tone. During severe episodes of protopathic pain, these autonomic pathways can
become activated as well and protopathic pains are often accompanied by nausea, vomiting, sweating, changes in vascular tone,
rapid heart rate, and so on. During his heart attack, for example,
my father was queasy, ashen faced, and sweating profusely.
Episodes of renal colic—the blockage of a kidney's outflow of

urine because of obstructing stones—typically cause intractable vomiting and sweating, and acute gallbladder disease behaves likewise. Epicritic pains, regardless of severity, rarely provoke autonomic outbursts.

Excluding ischemic pain, tubular blockages are a frequent cause of protopathic pain: kidney stones, gallstones, obstructed colons, blocked stomachs, narrowed urethras. Tubular structures like intestines, gall ducts, and ureters (the tubes connecting the kidney to the bladder) dilate behind points of obstruction as the unstoppable flow of stool, bile, or urine backs up like water behind a dam. As the stretched tubes struggle to expel the obstruction, a spasmodic cramping in the tube's muscular walls (colic) gives rise to waves of intense pain. Ironically, some of the most unbearable pains of human existence arise from these simple plumbing problems. If the natural force of muscular contractions cannot clear an obstruction, surgical methods must be used.

➤

Childbirth, carpal tunnel syndrome, and spinal discs may be uniquely human disorders, but not so the ancient pains of ischemia and colic. When we feel a pang in our chests or an ache in our bellies, our suffering dates back to the trilobites and beyond. Even dinosaurs had blocked colons. I know that this knowledge may be of little comfort to people about to have their gallbladders removed, their kidney stones sonicated, or their coronaries dilated with balloons. But the old adage holds that misery loves company, and, if that's true, we can take some solace in knowing that humans share protopathic pain with nearly every creature that has ever walked, crawled, wriggled, flown, or swam on the face of this good earth.

9

A MEGAPHONE SILENCED

Ricardo waddled on bent ankles into the clinic. He came for a refill of his seizure medications...and to relate a new problem. One of my retired colleagues had successfully removed a benign brain tumor from Ricardo's frontal lobe many years earlier, and I still saw the middle-aged Puerto Rican immigrant from time to time. Even though he suffered from yearly seizures, he rarely showed up at his scheduled office appointments. As I checked his record, I realized that I hadn't seen him for over two years and I was somewhat surprised at this sudden visit. Ricardo's new complaints proved to be stranger than his old ones. It wasn't his seizures that troubled him this time, but his legs. "No," he said, "they don't hurt." In fact, that was the problem. Ricardo no longer felt any pain in his legs at all.

A year earlier he had stepped on a nail at a construction site and didn't notice the wound until he removed his work boot later that evening. The nail had pierced the rubber sole and passed entirely through his foot. He should have been hobbled by pain, yet it felt only like he had a stone in his boot, nothing more. As an experiment, he tried pricking his other foot with a pin and felt nothing but a dull pressure, even when he drew blood. He wasn't completely numb; he could still feel something with his feet. He just couldn't feel pain.

The lack of pain sensation didn't bother him that much, and he forgot about the nail episode as soon as the wound healed. Then, months later, his sensation deteriorated further. In the weeks before he came to see me, he barely sensed his feet unless he looked at them or felt them with his hands. He had to watch his legs continuously as he walked, visually placing one foot in front of the other. Otherwise, he would trip and fall. In the dark he felt useless. When he couldn't see his legs clearly, they became like someone else's limbs, flailing out of his control. He could walk only by wrapping his hands around his thighs and manually guiding them forward.

Ricardo also noticed his ankles beginning to deform—very slightly at first, but now more dramatically. The ankles swelled at night and occasionally looked bruised and scraped, but still he knew no pain nor felt any tenderness in the traumatized joints. He came to the neurosurgery clinic with these odd complaints because we were the only doctors he knew and he had no place else to turn. Alas, his problem would have no surgical cure.

Like little Jimmy, the "boy who felt no pain" in Robert Marion's book, Ricardo had discovered nature's dark secret: pain isn't necessarily bad. Sometimes it's indispensable.

Marion's little Jimmy suffered from a congenital absence of his pain-sensing nerves, a genetic condition inherited from his father (who had a much milder form of the disease). Marion, a pediatric geneticist, first diagnosed the boy in infancy. When he revisited Jimmy three years later, Marion discovered a content toddler—who also happened to be missing the fingertips from both hands. Jimmy had bitten his nails down to poorly healing red stumps. Gruesome scars covered the boy, and he walked with a deformed, slapping gait. Incapable of feeling pain, Jimmy feared nothing and his battle-scarred body proved it.

Inherited sensory neuropathies as advanced as this are quite rare, but other, more common illnesses can produce a similar crippling reduction in pain sensibility. Hansen's disease, which still exists in developed countries, makes victims so impervious to pain that their noses, lips, hands, and feet can be literally worn away by repeated traumas. Named after nineteenth-century Norwegian physician Gerhard Hansen, the disease is caused by a mycobacterium, the same species of microbe responsible for tuberculosis. The more ubiquitous tubercle bacilli likes to invade the lungs, while Hansen's microbes prefer human peripheral nerves, invading and destroying them over time. Although few people recognize the eponymic name for this dreaded malady, everybody knows its Biblical name: leprosy, from the Greek *lepros* (scaly).

The deformities caused by mycobacterium leprae have been variously attributed to God's will, to animals eating insensate limbs as the afflicted slept, and to the disease simply rotting the flesh away. In truth, the deformities are the inevitable consequence of numbness, particularly numbness to pain, and can occur in any disease in which the sensation of pain is lost. Since they feel no pain, victims bite their lips, rub their noses, and chew their nails with such abandon that bodily tissue slowly erodes. By the age of three, little Jimmy had already lost part of his fingers and would certainly suffer more unintentional self-mutilation before he reached adulthood. The hands and feet of longtime diabetics and paralytics likewise become deformed and covered with pressure sores. Patients with trigeminal neuralgia who have their corneas rendered numb by alcohol nerve blocks will ultimately go blind from unchecked corneal scarring. When stripped of pain's discipline, we neglect our bodies until they become battered beyond recognition.

The skeletal joints also suffer the ravages of painlessness. All joints have a defined range of motion. If a joint travels beyond that range of motion, even by a few degrees, the ligaments surrounding the joint, called the joint's capsule, scream out with pain. No structural barriers prevent the knee and elbow joints from bending in the "wrong" direction; we simply won't allow the joints to bend contrary to their normal range of motion because it's too painful to do so (as anyone who has ever hyperextended a knee or elbow can verify). Without pain as a "brake," our joints will chronically deviate from their designed limits, resulting in joint damage. As we take each step, subtle pain sensations provide our muscles the information they need to keep the joints in correct alignment.

Joint sensitivity does have a negative side, in that it causes the pain of common osteoarthritis. As we age, the ligaments and limb muscles responsible for stabilizing our joints grow lax. The cartilage pads inside the joints begin to dry out and stiffen, a result of the same process that degenerates the discs within our spines. The bones surrounding the joint also deform with age, thanks to the continuous remodeling caused by decades of wear and tear. These changes all work together to distort and weaken aging joints, creating small degrees of joint instability. As an arthritic man walks, his hips and knees slide subtly beyond their intended range of motion, causing pain.

Joints provide auditory evidence of this instability. If a joint travels beyond its normal range too severely, the opposing bone surfaces will separate very slightly, creating a small vacuum that allows dissolved gases in the blood (mostly nitrogen) to bubble into the joint spaces. When the joint returns to its normal position, the separation vanishes and the gas bubbles pop, making a snapping noise similar to that made by imploding gas pockets in chewing gum. Some people can voluntarily distract their finger joints to achieve this gas-popping sound ("cracking the knuckles"); arthritic joints may crack even during normal activities. In severely affected joints, gas bubbles may be present all the time. For example, nitrogen bubbles are quite common on X-ray images of degenerated spinal joints. That's why most elderly people can feel or hear snapping in their spines on a daily basis.

Joint instability can happen over many years, as in the case of osteoarthritis, or in an instant. The anterior cruciate ligament (ACL) is a thick fibrous band lying at the center of the knee joint. The ACL anchors the thigh bone (femur) to the large shinbone (tibia) and prevents the femur from sliding forward as we walk. When a football player ruptures his ACL, he renders his knee immediately unstable. The team's trainers can detect this instability right on the playing field by bending the knee, grabbing behind the calf, and pulling the lower leg forward to see how much "give" they can elicit. Whether they realize it or not, ardent football fans have seen trainers perform this maneuver a hundred times. Even without an ACL, the injured player can get up and limp off the field. The joint won't fall apart, although the amount of pain generated by an acutely destabilized knee can be extreme.

When a joint is driven beyond its range of motion repeatedly, the smooth articulating surfaces of the adjoining bones can be stripped away, damaging the joint even more. Even after it heals, a knee without an ACL is prone to delayed problems because of the excessive slipping of the femur on the tibia. That's why professional athletes are so often hobbled and in pain during their later lives. With joints destabilized by injuries and aging muscles no longer able to compensate for loosening joints, they endure increased joint pain and accelerated joint wear.

A joint rendered insensitive to pain, however, suffers a worse fate than one wrecked by a single incident on a football field. The ancient Chinese employed a form of slow execution called "the death of a thousand cuts" in which the victim was sliced repeatedly with a knife. Each individual wound was superficial and nonlethal, but the accumulation of hundreds of these cuts proved fatal. The insensate joint dies a similar protracted death, damaged by a thousand injuries delivered over months. Ricardo's ankles were in the midst of this slow execution.

Since he couldn't feel pain in his legs any longer and couldn't even tell the position of his feet, Ricardo sprained his ankles with every step. On one occasion he entered a bright room from a darkened hallway and, as he looked down, was horrified to find that he had been walking on the outsides of his ankles, with his feet turned inward. No wonder his ankles looked swollen and bruised all the time. Eventually his ankle ligaments would be stretched hopelessly out of shape, the bones cracked and their cartilage sanded away. The joints would then fuse into amorphous lumps...and all without a lick of pain.

Joints destroyed by a lack of normal painful feedback are called Charcot's joints, after the nineteenth-century French neurologist who first described them, Jean Charcot. Charcot's joints occur in a variety of diseases, including Hansen's disease, congenital neuropathies, multiple sclerosis, spinal cord injuries, and strokes. The classic cause of Charcot's joints—and at one time the most common cause—is a disease known as tabes dorsalis, Latin for "a wasting of the back."

In tabes, the back, or dorsal, part of the spinal cord wastes away. The sensory pathways reside in this area; the front (ventral) cord containing the motor fibers is immune to the disease and victims of tabes rarely experience gross weakness. Tabes, like Hansen's disease, is the handiwork of a microbe with a taste for nerve fibers: treponema pallidum. Also like Hansen's disease, infection with treponema pallidum carries a far more familiar moniker: syphilis (named after a fictional shepherd in the Fracastorius poem "Syphilis sive Morbus Gallicus").

Ricardo admitted having a case of syphilis in his younger and "wilder" days but thought he had been treated adequately. Testing of his spinal fluid proved him right on the first count but mistaken on the second. He now had tertiary syphilis and a few Charcot's joints to go along with it. Medical therapy would stop the disease, save his life, and prevent more misery in the future. Some of his sensation might even return, but his deformed ankles would linger forever. Ricardo's bent ankles, like little Jimmy's stumplike fingers, serve as reminders of those good things that pain does for us. The next time a shoulder groans or a knee aches, remember what would happen if we felt no pain at all. We would very quickly have no shoulders or knees at all. Old and painful joints are preferable to joints worn to uselessness in our youths by unperceived traumas. Or, in the words of the Bard (from *2 Henry IV*):

> *I were better eaten to death with a rust than to be scoured to nothing with perpetual motion.*

Those who wish for a pain-free existence—be careful what you wish for; read Professor Marion's account and wish again.

We need the megaphone.

10

A TWILIGHT BETWEEN SLEEP AND DEATH

*Gentleman, I have seen something today
that will go around the world.*

—surgeon Henry Bigelow, after
witnessing the first demonstration of
general anesthesia in 1846

Bob, our chief cardiothoracic resident, hustled to the intensive care unit at my request. I was an inexperienced surgical intern at the time and I knew that Mr. Lattimer's problem was out of my control. I needed help, and fast.

Mr. Lattimer, a sixty-seven-year-old banker, had undergone routine coronary artery bypassing two days earlier and had been doing quite well. The critical care physician weaned him from his endotracheal breathing tube the morning after surgery; Mr. Lattimer even managed a lunch of low-salt chicken soup shortly thereafter. Forty-eight hours later the patient still looked alert and comfortable. I yanked the drainage tubes from his chest and was about to send him out of the ICU when he became acutely short of breath.

Right before my eyes, Mr. Lattimer began to struggle for air and his lips turned dark. He began clutching his chest, clawing at the white gauze that still covered his fresh chest wound. I asked the nurses to summon Bob as I placed an oxygen mask on Mr.

Lattimer's face. Sweat now beaded on the man's distressed brow. My mind raced. Was he having a heart attack? Perhaps a pulmonary embolism?

Fortunately, Bob was on the next floor and arrived within minutes. "What's wrong here, sport?"

"Mr. Lattimer." I pointed to the gasping man. "He can't breathe."

"Let's have a look."

Bob joined me at the bedside and we watched together as Mr. Lattimer's blood pressure plummeted. One twenty. One hundred. Ninety. Bob glanced up at the blood pressure tracing on the electrical monitor just above Mr. Lattimer's bed.

"Uh-oh. Look." Bob pointed to the tracing. "He has a paradoxical pulse." Bob referred to the exaggerated manner in which the patient's blood pressure rose and fell with his respirations. I didn't know much at the time, but I knew what a paradoxical pulse meant: Mr. Lattimer was bleeding into his chest. One of the stitches in his heart must have unraveled, perhaps due to the force of the chest tubes being removed, and now this leaking blood threatened to smother his heart, a condition known as cardiac tamponade. Tamponade kills a postoperative heart patient in minutes. We had no time to get him to an operating room.

"Here, sport." Bob threw a yellow ICU gown at me and grabbed one for himself. "If you value your clothes, put that on. You'll need it. Now, give me a hand." Bob yelled for the nurses to summon an anesthesiologist, stat.

I pulled the dressings from Mr. Lattimer's wounds while Bob gloved his hands. Bob then quickly uncapped a large bottle of iodine solution and dumped the brown liquid on the man's heaving chest. Mr. Lattimer was at this moment barely conscious, his eyes closed and his lips silently forming the words "Help me" over and over. Opening a small pack of instruments we kept taped to every heart patient's bed for just such an occasion, Bob used them to tear the skin staples from the wound and pulled the skin edges apart, exposing the sternum beneath.

"Here, Frank. Hold this open."

I grabbed the skin edges and pulled. With four deft snips of his wire cutter, Bob loosened the sterum and inserted his fingers between the freshly sawed edges of bone. Yanking hard, he opened the chest cavity and, in doing so, unleashed a torrent of black blood. This old blood was soon followed by a pulsatile stream of fresher red blood that shot over Bob's shoulder and splattered on the wall behind him. The pericardial sac had been disrupted by the bleeding, and we could easily see Mr. Lattimer's heart twisting and splashing within his open chest. Bob traced the stream of fresh blood to a small hole in the aorta—one of the new vein grafts had detached from the body's main artery, exposing an open rent. Cupping his hand around the massive vessel, Bob squeezed and halted the bleeding; he called again for the nurses to notify the operating room. We now had the situation under temporary control.

With the tamponade relieved, Mr. Lattimer's blood pressure shot back up to normal and his breathing became less labored. Renewed with oxygenated blood, the banker immediately woke and, upon gazing down at his exposed heart, began screaming at the top of his lungs. Although I found his screaming eminently justified, the noise filled the room with an unnerving noise bordering on the horrible. Another surgical resident showed up to hold the hysterical patient's head down so that he couldn't see what was going on, and a nurse astutely tossed a sterile towel across the bloodied chest. None of this helped. The poor man bucked and struggled mightily. Bob did his best to hang on to the fragile aorta, but soon we were all a soggy reddened mess. The situation began to look more like an Aztec sacrifice than a heroic lifesaving measure.

Fortunately, an anesthesiologist arrived to put us all out of our misery. "No problem." He grinned. "We'll fix this in a jiffy." He infused a mixture of lorazapam and ketamine into Mr. Lattimer's jugular venous line, instantly rendering him unconscious. After another infusion, this time of the paralytic drug curare, the patient's body fell totally flaccid, allowing the anesthesiologist to glide a breathing tube effortlessly into his windpipe. We could now take Mr. Lattimer back to the operating room at our leisure.

"He won't remember a thing!" The anesthesiologist beamed.

"How can he forget seeing his own heart?" I asked, somewhat unconvinced. The anesthesiologist held up his now-empty syringes of drugs.

"A little dissociative anesthesia, my friend. Modern mind control. I'm telling you, he won't remember a thing. Trust me."

We repaired the hole in Mr. Lattimer's aorta, and this time the postoperative recovery went without a hitch. Just before we discharged him, I asked Mr. Lattimer how he enjoyed his stay in the hospital.

"Oh, great. A very nice place. In fact, this whole experience has been better than I could have imagined. Except for that nasty thing in the ICU."

"What nasty thing?"

"That low-salt chicken soup. Who ever heard of low-salt chicken soup? I don't think I could tolerate that stuff again."

I have no doubt that at some time in the years following his surgery, Mr. Lattimer awakened in a cold sweat, convinced that he had been witness to the beating of his own heart. He then wondered if it was truly a bad dream. *Boy,* he must have thought, *I shouldn't eat stuffed peppers before going to bed. It all seemed so darned real...*

The miracle of anesthesia.

➤

At one time surgeons weren't doctors but barbers. Or tradesmen. Or butchers. Or whoever else a real physician could dupe, cajole, or bribe into performing an operation. Skill and education were superfluous for the "surgeons" of antiquity. Prior to the advent of anesthesia, the only things surgeons really needed were strong assistants and a strong stomach: strong assistants to hold down struggling patients, and a strong stomach to put up with their horrific outcries. A surgeon's repertoire was limited to procedures that could be done crudely and swiftly: limb amputations, suturing of lacerations, dental extractions, and, for the exceptionally bold, mastectomies and jaw resections for cancer. Operating inside the chest, head, or abdomen proved impossible since there were no reliable means of sedating the patient for several hours. Consequently, such operations were rarely attempted.

Surgeon and noted author Richard Selzer provided one of the best descriptions of how a major operation looked and felt in the days prior to general anesthesia. In his book *Raising the Dead,* Selzer recounts the brutal resection of a large chest wall cancer from famed novelist Fanny d'Arblay. (Warning: The details of d'Arblay's operation aren't for the fainthearted.) Selzer's account gives modern readers an idea of why they should give thanks to the inventors of anesthesia.

Early attempts at anesthesia now seem as crude as the surgical procedures themselves. Ancient Assyrians strangulated infants into unconsciousness before performing ritual circumcisions. Some cultures used blows to the head to induce a semblance of anesthesia, a practice now seen only in cartoons and Three Stooges films. Ancient physicians also encouraged the smoking of hemp or hashish prior to surgery, or rendered their patients stuporous with opium or wine (contrary to popular belief, however, alcohol is a poor analgesic). In the Middle Ages surgeons held a sponge soaked with medicinal herbs over the patient's face (the "soporific sponge of Theodoric"). French surgeon Dupuytren had a particularly novel approach—he once insulted a woman until she passed out, then proceeded to operate.

The modern history of anesthesia begins with legendary chemist (and discoverer of oxygen) Joseph Priestly. Priestly synthesized the first practical anesthetic gas—nitrous oxide—in the late 1700s, although he never used it for medicinal purposes. Instead, nitrous oxide became the recreational intoxicant du jour for the well-to-do, who promptly dubbed it "laughing gas." Sir Humphrey Davy, another famous chemist of the same era, marveled at how partygoers under the influence of laughing gas felt little or no pain. He suggested giving nitrous oxide to surgical patients and even tried a few experiments on his own body to prove his point, but his brilliant proposal fell on deaf ears. Decades would pass before medical science rediscovered the value of nitrous oxide and other sedative gases.

In the 1840s physicians again became interested in nitrous oxide and a related compound, ether. Like nitrous oxide, ether started out as a recreational drug (there's always been a fine line between useful analgesics and dangerous recreational drugs, a point we will revisit later). Valerius Cordus discovered ether

("sweet oil of vitriol") in 1540; later that same year Swiss alchemist Paracelsus added it to his chicken feed and was astounded when all of his chickens passed out. Ether had its first
medical application during the late 1700s, when it was used
to treat colic. In 1796 physicians again discovered that deep inhalation of ether produces profound sleep (the chickens of
Paracelsus having been long forgotten), but they considered the
substance too toxic for therapeutic use.

In 1818 Faraday inhaled a mixture of ether vapors and oxygen and experienced a pleasant intoxication similar to that
produced by alcohol and laughing gas. Aware of Faraday's observations, medical students began organizing ether parties,
called "jags," akin to the beer keg parties I attended as a student.
One physician in attendance at an ether jag was Dr. Crawford
Long, a country surgeon hailing from Jefferson, Georgia. As
Davy had observed with nitrous oxide years before, Long found
that revelers staggering about under the influence of ether often
endured bodily injury without feeling pain. He became keenly
interested in ether as a clinical painkiller and in March 1842 ex-
cised a growth from the neck of a friend using ether inhalation.
The friend went along with the experiment in exchange for a reduced surgical fee. Long went on to apply ether anesthesia successfully on several more occasions. Unfortunately, Long lived far
from the major medical centers of his day and never bothered to
report his findings to the medical community at large. He would
later regret this.

At the same time Long was experimenting with ether, a free-
lance chemist named Colton roamed the New England countryside charging local residents twenty-five cents apiece to try
laughing gas. Colton possessed a dramatic flair and his demon-
strations had a circuslike atmosphere. His advertisements

proclaimed that several burly men would have to attend each demonstration to prevent those intoxicated by the gas from injuring themselves or others. During one fateful demonstration held at Hartford, Connecticut, in the winter of 1844, a young clerk named Cooley sniffed a bit of Colton's gas and immediately became so combative that he had to be subdued by the hired strong men. During the ensuing struggle, Cooley gashed his leg on a chair but didn't notice the wound until some minutes later—when nitrous oxide's effect wore off.

Hartford's dentist at the time, Dr. Horace Wells, witnessed this curious event and after the demonstration concluded, closely interrogated the injured clerk, who assured Wells that he had indeed felt no pain under the influence of laughing gas. That evening Wells allowed himself to be put to sleep under nitrous oxide. The following morning he had one of his own teeth extracted as he breathed laughing gas administered by Colton. He felt no pain at all. Elated by his discovery, Wells began using the gas in his own practice and soon arranged a public demonstration of his "painless dentistry" for a group of Harvard medical students and professors at the Massachusetts General Hospital in Boston.

The well-publicized demonstration took place in January 1845. Wells administered laughing gas to his selected patient and proceeded to extract the man's infected tooth. Unfortunately, the dose of gas Wells gave him proved inadequate and the patient began yelling in pain. With no apparatus to control the amount of nitrous oxide entering his patient's lungs, Wells could not predict the level of analgesia, and in this instance he fell short of achieving general anesthesia. A few of Wells's colleagues had warned him about this potential difficulty; one even urged him to use ether vapors instead, arguing that ether would be technically simpler to regulate. For some unknown reason, Wells rejected ether and proceeded with the laughing gas demonstration as planned.

As the patient bucked and yelped in the dentist's chair, medical students in attendance booed and hissed at the crestfallen Wells. Deeply humiliated, he gave up dentistry and committed suicide by cutting his own femoral artery three years later. Despondent over the botched demonstration, Wells died addicted to chloroform and under indictment for throwing acid at a prostitute. If his demise sounds like an overreaction to failure, remember that Wells had been convinced that his discovery would make him a legend (if he had followed his friend's advice and used ether, he would have succeeded). Going so quickly from hero to laughingstock proved too much for him to bear emotionally. In one of medical history's great ironies, his patient later confessed that he recalled feeling no pain during the extraction, despite his outcries. Wells had, in fact, succeeded.

Wells's former practice partner, Dr. William T. G. Morton of Boston, continued the search for painless dentistry. The joint dental practice of Wells and Morton had broken up years earlier because of financial difficulties, but Morton never lost his enthusiasm for nitrous oxide. After witnessing the public failure of nitrous oxide firsthand, however, Morton turned his attention to the substance Wells had rejected: ether.

At the time, Morton was working his way through Harvard Medical School by practicing dentistry on the side. One of his professors at Harvard, chemist Charles Jackson, had on one occasion rendered himself senseless by accidentally breathing fumes of sulfuric ether and had related this experience to Morton, who was deeply impressed. At least this was the story Jackson told years later, as he was trying to convince the scientific community of his own role in discovering anesthesia. After practicing on his own dog, Morton used ether on a patient to ease a difficult tooth extraction, with great success. Morton then petitioned Dr. John Warren (the same Harvard surgeon who presided over the Wells fiasco) to permit a public demonstration of a new kind of surgical pain control. Morton, undeterred by the embarrassing failure of nitrous oxide, had a plan much grander than that of his former partner. Unlike Wells, he wouldn't settle for a simple dental extraction. He wanted to prove his technique on a bona fide surgical procedure. Warren agreed, even though Morton never told him exactly what he planned to do. Given that Morton was only a second-year medical student at the time, Warren's consent seems somewhat foolhardy in retrospect. For whatever reason (perhaps because surgeons were willing to try anything at that point), Warren trusted Morton—and the rest, as they say, is history.

What happened on the day of Morton's demonstration—October 16, 1846—has passed into the realm of medical folklore. Bothered by last-minute technical problems, Morton showed up fifteen minutes late for the operation and Warren almost made the incision without him. When Morton finally arrived, Warren pointed to his quaking patient, Gilbert Abbott, and said icily, "Well, sir, your patient awaits you." Morton administered the ether, then pointed to the unconscious man and replied, "Doctor, *your* patient is ready." Warren proceeded to carve a benign tumor from Abbott's jaw in five minutes, eliciting nary a peep from the slumbering patient. The cadre of muscle men hired to restrain Abbott during the ordeal sat idly by and the room fell oppressively silent, an oddity for nineteenth-century operating theaters. After Abbott awakened dazed but unharmed, an amazed Warren turned at once to his stunned audience and uttered one of history's great understatements:

"Gentlemen, this is no humbug."

Today the "ether dome" used for this event remains a historic monument at Harvard Medical School. Dr. Oliver Wendell Holmes, the physician and renowned author, was so inspired by Morton's demonstration that he penned a letter to the medical student a few weeks after the event to propose a name for the new discovery. "The state," wrote Holmes, referring to the condition of Morton's etherized patient, "should, I think, be called 'anaesthesia.'" Holmes correctly predicted that his word would quickly enter the lexicon of every civilized nation.

Instead of becoming a celebrity, Morton damaged his reputation by patenting ether for his own financial gain, a grave error that yielded only years of acrimonious debate. (He would later redeem himself by administering ether to thousands of soldiers during the Civil War.) To protect his patent priority, Morton failed to identify his anesthetic drug as ether, instead calling it "letheon" and implying that it was his own invention. Many in attendance at the first demonstration of "letheon" guessed that it contained ether because of the smell, but Morton refused to identify the substance. Morton's apologists later argued that this deception was Morton's way of preventing others from using ether before he had worked out certain safety issues. More cynical observers noted that Morton was, after all, a dentist, and that dentists of that era would patent water if they thought they could get away with it. Many were offended that so awesome a discovery could be copyrighted for the use and enrichment of a single man. Upon discovering that letheon was, in fact, ordinary sulfuric ether, several people contested Morton's patent, among them: Crawford Long, the Georgian surgeon who first successfully used ether four years before Morton's demonstration, and Charles Jackson, the chemistry professor who suggested ether to Morton.

Morton and his allies fought back, criticizing Long for his

failure to report his findings and alleging that Jackson was little more than an ignorant opportunist who had contributed nothing of value to the discovery. Allegations of ethical impropriety flew back and forth, but in the end Long never received proper credit during his lifetime. Jackson went insane at Morton's grave after seeing an inscription giving Morton sole credit for the discovery of ether and later died in an asylum. And Morton succumbed to a stroke at the age of forty-eight, ending his career a bitter, bankrupt man. He was bankrupt largely because of the jealous Jackson, who spent the latter half of his life trying to ruin his old student. The ether controversy so consumed Morton that he abandoned the final two years of his medical degree at Harvard. The father of anesthesiology never even managed to become a licensed physician. His dental practice failed and his attempt to make a windfall from an ether inhalation device collapsed after customers realized they could simply make the devices themselves.

Morton's patent struggle started a controversy that has never been fully resolved. Although it is currently acceptable to patent a drug or piece of medical equipment, patenting a medical or surgical procedure (like the controlled administration of ether to induce sleep) remains impossible even today. Ethicists argue that it's unfair to license a lifesaving procedure that should be the intellectual property of humankind at large, but I find it unclear why the same argument doesn't apply to proprietary ownership of lifesaving drugs like AZT (the AIDS drug). Despite his legal woes, Morton's place in the pantheon of modern medicine remains secure. His tombstone justly reads: "THE INVENTOR AND REVEALER OF ANESTHETIC INHALATION. BEFORE WHOM, IN ALL TIME, SURGERY WAS AGONY..."

Colton, the peripatetic chemist and occasional showman,

never gave up on nitrous oxide. In the 1860s, armed with better technology, he reintroduced laughing gas into the practice of dentistry, where it remains to the present day. In fact, of all the drugs used in the early days of general anesthesia, only nitrous oxide remains in daily use.

After the success of ether, the search was on for better anesthetic agents, ones that didn't smell quite so awful. Next came chloroform, a gentler anesthetic first used in 1847 by Scottish obstetrician James Young Simpson for easing the pain of labor. Unfortunately, volatile substances like ether and chloroform have a tendency to burn or even explode. Operating rooms quickly became hazardous places for doctors and patients alike. After the introduction of electric cauterization by American brain surgeon Harvey Cushing in the first half of this century, ether and other explosive anesthetics became even more problematic. The slightest electric spark in a room filled with ether vapor could reduce an entire hospital wing to smoking rubble. As operating rooms entered the electrical age, ether and chloroform became liabilities and were soon banned in favor of safer gases like halothane and, of course, nitrous oxide. Despite their dangers, these agents enjoyed nearly a century of use and eased the suffering of countless thousands.

❧

The next big advance in general anesthesia involved the control of respiration in sleeping patients. Since antiquity, surgeons have known that the best patient is an unconscious one. Making someone unconscious turns out to be relatively easy—that much has been known for centuries. Keeping them unconscious for hours and safely reviving them later—that proves to be a significantly more difficult task. Ancient physicians recognized that strangulation, bonks on the head, and ingesting large amounts of opium or fermented beverages could knock a person out cold, but they didn't know how to control the length of time the victim would stay unconscious, nor could they guarantee that patients who were choked, beaten, drugged, or (in the weird case of Dupuytren) berated into utter senselessness would awaken with all their faculties...or awaken at all. In fact, many didn't awaken. Soporifics like opium, barbiturates, and alcohol can cause fatal respiratory depression at the doses needed to achieve complete insensibility to pain. Without some artificial means of maintaining respiration, patients held unconscious under the influence of these drugs will asphyxiate before any operation could be completed.

Narcotics and alcohol also stimulate vomiting. This invites disaster in lethargic patients prone to inhaling highly acidic stomach contents into their delicate lungs. This lethal event, now known as aspiration, remains a problem even today (it's why surgical patients should not eat anything during the hours prior to general anesthesia).

Ether, on the other hand, could render patients unconscious without severely depressing their respiratory drive. This made it quite useful at a time when artificial respiration was unknown. Ether anesthesia was far from perfect, however. The patient might still vomit or abruptly stop breathing, and if that happened, the ether assistant could do little except watch as the patient expired.

Around the turn of the century, physicians developed ways of preventing aspiration and controlling respiration. At first, assistants used rubber face masks placed tightly over the patient's mouth and nose. By squeezing a balloon attached to the mask, the assistant could inflate the lungs manually. This method worked for short periods, but it also had a tendency to inflate the stomach as well as the lungs, increasing the risk of vomiting. Later, anesthesia assistants began inserting metal breathing tubes directly into the windpipes of anesthetized patients. These tubes served a dual purpose: they blocked vomit from entering the lungs and provided a more direct conduit for artificially ventilating patients who had ceased to breathe on their own. Today such endotracheal tubes (or ET tubes as they are now called) are made of plastic. With the advent of ET tubes and the later invention of mechanized ventilators, anesthesiologists could utilize any number of drugs to induce a pharmacologic coma—scopolamine, Pentothal, morphine—without fear of asphyxiation.

By the middle of this century, artificial ventilation alone could maintain adequate oxygenation in a human being. Muscular effort on the part of the anesthetized patient was no longer needed. Physicians could now transiently paralyze patients in addition to rendering them unconscious. Why would anesthesiologists want to paralyze patients temporarily? For one thing, paralysis makes the chest wall more compliant, allowing more efficient mechanical ventilation. Furthermore, it facilitates operating within cavities like the abdomen and chest, since the surgeon no longer has to wrestle the patient's own muscular tone to hold the cavity open. Finally, it provides a margin of safety during delicate operations on the brain, spinal cord, and eyes. Even under ether or barbiturate anesthesia, patients may abruptly move without warning, a disastrous occurrence during delicate stages of an operation. By chemically paralyzing Mr. Lattimer, the anesthesiologist could control his airway and breathe for him with ease. The anesthesiologist could have simply put Mr. Lattimer to sleep, but even under general anesthesia, he still might have choked and gagged on the ET tube.

To produce chemical paralysis, anesthesiologists turned to an Amazonian plant poison known since the days of Sir Walter Raleigh: curare. South American Indians coated their arrows with this toxin; minuscule amounts rendered their prey paralyzed and unable to breathe, and death from asphyxiation followed within minutes. In the 1930s physicians used tiny doses of curare to ease the spasms of tetanus and to "calm" mentally ill patients. In the 1940s curare moved into the operating room. Today anesthesiologists use curare derivatives or similar paralytic drugs, notably succinylcholine, in virtually every case of general anesthesia.

➤

In the early 1900s the specialty of anesthesia still consisted of poorly trained assistants dripping ether onto a patient's mouth. Save for occasionally feeling the pulse, the ether assistant paid little attention to the patient's vital signs. In truth, assistants barely looked at the patient at all. Cushing, the aforementioned coinventor of electric cautery, changed this by introducing blood pressure monitoring into the operating room. He also came up with another ingenius idea: the anesthesia record. Cushing asked his anesthesia assistants to measure pulse, blood pressure, and respiratory rate of his patients every five minutes and to graph these numbers on a piece of paper during the operation. He also asked them to record when the operation began and ended, how much blood was lost, how much ether or other anesthetic drugs were administered, and other significant facts concerning the case. Modern anesthesiologists keep records very similar to the one first designed by Cushing ninety years ago.

The introduction of endotracheal tubes, better monitoring devices, and newer anesthetic drugs mandated the creation of anesthesiology as a formal specialty. No longer could general anesthesia be entrusted to a nurse or intern with little specific training or experience. A Board of Anesthesiology was created, and today's anesthesiologists must now spend four or five years in postgraduate training before they are licensed to administer general anesthetics. Likewise, nurse anesthetists intensively study the physiology and pharmacology of anesthesia, and must serve apprenticeships in the operating room before becoming certified nurse anesthetists (CNAs).

By the end of the twentieth century, an anesthesiologist's armamentarium contained hundreds of drugs: drugs to induce sleep, to induce paralysis, to raise and lower blood pressure, to ease pain, to raise and lower heart rate, to correct aberrant heart rhythms, to regulate blood sugar, to increase urine output, and so on. A patient undergoing major surgery will now have a temperature probe in the rectum to measure core body temperature; a catheter in the radial artery at the wrist to measure blood pressure; a bladder catheter to collect and measure urine output; a nasogastric tube to keep the stomach decompressed; an endotracheal tube; a large intravenous line in the jugular vein to instill drugs and intravenous fluids and also to monitor the central venous pressure; an echocardiographic probe in the esophagus to visualize the beating heart and measure cardiac output; electrodes on the scalp to measure brain function; electrodes on the arm to judge how well the paralytic drugs are working; a pulse oximeter on the index finger to measure how much oxygen is circulating in the blood; electrocardiographic leads taped to the chest wall to record heart rhythms; and, finally, defibrillator paddles glued to the chest to provide a shock should defibrillation occur. In addition, the patient rests on a blanket that can be heated or cooled to regulate body temperature; the endotracheal tube also contains a computerized device to measure the concentration of oxygen, carbon dioxide, and anesthetic gases flowing in and out of the lungs. The net result of this impressive pharmacological and technological array? The ability to anesthetize almost anyone, no matter how ill, with a mortality rate of less than one in every ten thousand operations (compared to about one death in every five or ten operations at the turn of the century).

General anesthesia ranks high among the greatest achievements of our age. Without it, surgery would still consist largely of amputations. The story of surgery has been written mostly by anesthesiologists, not by surgeons. Liver transplantation, heart bypassing, and brain tumor extirpations are great feats but would be impossible in awake patients, no matter how skilled the surgeon may be.

And the story of anesthesia has been largely written by dentists, as difficult as that may be for medical doctors to swallow. The reason for the dominance of dentists in this field may have been economic. Since early physicians didn't profit directly from surgical procedures, they had little incentive to make surgery palatable for patients. Moreover, a patient with a gangrenous leg has but one alternative to surgery: death. Thus, barber-surgeons were guaranteed a supply of patients, no matter how foul their methods may have been. Dentists, on the other hand, were in a more difficult situation financially. They made their living doing purely elective procedures, and few people elected to have root canals or extractions without something to dull their pain. Consequently, the average dentist, preanesthesia, had little to do. A dentist who had a proprietary way of making dentistry painless could become very busy—and very rich.

The next time we are confronted with a large bill from our dentists, we can take comfort in knowing that greedy dentists gave us general anesthesia and that general anesthesia gave us modern surgery. Were it not for dentists, anesthesia might still consist of a rag stuffed into our mouths and a set of strong hands on our arms and legs.

➤

Not all surgical procedures require an unconscious patient. Many procedures can be accomplished in awake patients after numbing the appropriate part of the body, a technique called local anesthesia. Local anesthesia had its origins in antiquity. Incan shamans of the twelfth century performed trephinations on headache victims, cutting wide holes into the skull with flint knives to permit evil spirits to escape. After slicing open the scalp, shamans chewed coca leaves and spit into the wounds. Cocaine dissolved in their saliva served to deaden the pain.

Scientists first purified cocaine from the coca plant in 1860. Twenty years later a physician named Von Anrep injected it under his skin and found that it eliminated the pain of pinpricks. Despite this finding, no one considered cocaine as a useful drug until ten years after Von Anrep's experiment. It was championed next by two young (but influential) Viennese physicians, Karl Koller, and another man who would later make something of a name for himself outside the field of pharmacology—Sigmund Freud.

Freud, not surprisingly, was most interested in the effect of cocaine on behavior. Koller, on the other hand, appreciated the anesthetic properties of the drug and introduced it into ophthalmology for use in eye surgery. A short time later, in 1884, Hall introduced it into dentistry, and a year after that, the legendary surgeon William Halstead used injectable cocaine to produce "nerve blocks" for limb surgery. At about the same time that Halstead was experimenting with regional anesthesia, Corning proposed injecting cocaine directly into the spinal fluid—the birth of spinal anesthesia.

Cocaine has one serious drawback: it's highly addictive. In addition to providing anesthesia, cocaine taken systemically causes a pleasurable sensation that users find habit forming. Freud tried to exploit cocaine's psychoactive properties to wean patients from morphine addiction but only succeeded in creating the world's first cocaine addicts instead. Even the fictional Sherlock Holmes wrestled with cocaine dependency. Addiction plagued patients and physicians alike, and some famous researchers—including Halstead—succumbed to cocaine's allure. Pharmacologists at the turn of the century began searching for a cocaine substitute that would have the anesthetic properties of the drug minus the psychological side effects. In 1905 Einhorn created the first cocaine substitute: procaine. Procaine was marketed under the trade name Novocain and was an instant success. Unfortunately, many patients developed life-threatening allergies to the drug and it has now been replaced with the hypoallergenic drug lidocaine. Although no longer used, Novocain's legacy lives on. Today most people still generically refer to all local anesthetics as Novocain.

How do anesthetic drugs work to relieve pain? We have learned a great deal about the mechanism of action of these drugs, but not all questions have been answered. We now know how local anesthetics like cocaine, procaine, and lidocaine work, but general anesthetics like ether and nitrous oxide remain more mysterious.

Local anesthetics block the transmission of electrical impulses along peripheral nerves. Nerve cells act like little batteries by pumping electrically charged atoms known as ions—specifically potassium and sodium ions—across their membranes to create an electric field. This field can be used to conduct nerve signals. Local anesthetics weaken the nerve's ion-pumping action and eliminate the electric field, rendering the nerve cell temporarily inoperative. The paralysis of nerve function affects both motor and sensory nerves equally, explaining why patients under spinal anesthesia have neither motion or sensation in their legs.

Because they act on an organ considerably more complicated than a nerve, namely the brain, general anesthetics have proven harder to decipher. Some anesthetics, like barbiturates, cause unconsciousness by inhibiting all of the nerve cells of the brain at once. Others, like ether and nitrous oxide, appear only to affect the sleep centers in the brain stem.

I hesitate to call the state induced by ether and other inhalational agents "sleep." In fact, as the title of this chapter suggests, general anesthesia is more of a twilight state hovering between sleep and brain death. (Using barbiturate anesthesia, patients can even be made to look brain-dead, complete with a "flat-line" EEG.) If I am asleep on my couch and someone starts sawing my leg off, I will rapidly awaken (hopefully). If I am under ether anesthesia, I will not. Drugs like ether not only create a sleeplike state, they also disconnect the sleep state from the arousal mechanisms that govern normal sleep. Exactly how they do this remains unclear.

Even more mysterious are the dissociative drugs like keta-mine. These agents disconnect, or dissociate, patients from their pain. As in the case of Mr. Lattimer, they can also make patients "forget" a painful experience.

Prior to the invention of antipsychotic drugs in the 1950s, psychiatrists used a now-discredited operation known as frontal lobotomy to "quiet" their more difficult patients. The most popular version of the operation was performed with an ice pick. The operator inserted an ice pick under the upper eyelids and hit the pick with a small mallet to drive it into the frontal lobes. The operator then rotated the pick vigorously to destroy both lobes. This created a docile, albeit somewhat dull, patient.

The inventor of lobotomy, Portuguese neurologist António Egas Moniz (who received a Nobel Prize for this dubious creation, believe it or not), theorized that lobotomy disrupted the patient's perception of psychic pain. That may or may not have been true, but what couldn't be disputed was how some lobotomized patients seemed disconnected from their physical pain. Patients previously afflicted with cancer pain, for example, seemed oblivious to it after extensive lobotomies. When asked about their pain, they simply smiled and replied, "Oh yes, it's still there," but they no longer thought it was a bad thing. This observation prompted some surgeons to use lobotomy for pain control alone in terminally ill patients, and a modified version of the procedure (known as cingulotomy) is still performed for that purpose on rare occasions.

The lobotomy experience taught neuroscientists that it's possible to dissociate the physical sensation of pain from the emotional perception of pain as unpleasant. Lobotomized patients still felt pain; they just didn't let it bother them anymore. Pharmacologists soon figured out ways to achieve this effect temporarily with drugs. Under dissociative anesthesia, the patient may be awake and receiving no analgesia, yet the sensations he or she feels aren't perceived as unpleasant.

When administered after the event, these drugs can also render a patient amnesic, with no recollection of the painful event at all. Mr. Lattimar couldn't recall anything that happened to him during his first stay in the ICU, save for the crummy chicken soup. The anesthesiologist chose the drugs he gave Mr. Lattimer precisely for that purpose. The power of these drugs to erase our memories raises an interesting ethical and philosophical question: If we can't remember pain, did it really occur? It's a modified version of the old "If a tree falls in the forest..." dilemma.

Technically, all we really need to perform painless surgery are two drugs: a paralytic agent to keep patients from yelling and wriggling about during the operation and an amnesic agent administered afterward to make them forget what terrible thing we just did to them. Without any anesthesia save curare, paralyzed patients will be in silent agony during the operation itself, of course, since they will be feeling everything while incapable of moving a muscle in protest. The thought of having open-heart surgery while fully awake and totally paralyzed must rank as one of the most awful images the average intellect can conjure. Nevertheless, with the appropriate amnesic agent, we wouldn't remember any of it, so why should it matter?

In fact, in certain select pediatric cases, anesthesiologists may use only drug-induced paralysis. They may not even use amnesic drugs afterward—babies can't remember anything, anyway. I had a spinal tap without anesthesia as an infant and I don't recall a thing. I'm sure I screamed bloody murder at the time, but it hasn't affected me otherwise.

This may sound cruel, but in critically ill adults and very tiny infants, anesthetic drugs may carry more risk than amnesic drugs. Ironically, the anesthesiologist often *wants* the patient to be in some degree of discomfort during the case. The drugs used to induce anesthesia often cause the blood pressure to drop dangerously low, and my anesthesiologists sometimes implore me to "hurry up and hurt this person" so that the blood pressure and pulse rate will rise in response to a painful stimulus. Patients, of course, have no memory of this. Our goal isn't to make every moment of surgery pain free in an absolute sense, but to exit the operating room with a live patient, one who—like Mr. Lattimer—believes that the operation, perceived as a whole, was a wonderful experience.

I'm a bit of a wimp. I hate to see people in pain. There are occasions when I have to put in a skin stitch or a staple and, for technical reasons, I can't use even the tiniest bit of local anesthesia (for example, when closing a small wound near the site of a previous brain operation—a small amount of lidocaine coming into direct contact with the brain may cause death). Even inflicting that small amount of pain on an awake patient makes me uncomfortable. Brain surgeons do almost all of their operations under general anesthesia and that may be one reason I went into neurosurgery at all. One of my old teachers used to say: "If it can't be done under general anesthesia, the patient doesn't need it anyway."

I simply cannot fathom life as a surgeon-barber prior to the 1840s. The thought of slicing a limb from a writhing, screaming patient appalls me. I can't imagine a world without general anesthesia, lidocaine, or morphine. Modern patients cannot know what a great debt they owe to those greedy, squabbling dentists.

Amazingly, some religious groups of the nineteenth century opposed general anesthesia, saying it was God's will for us to suffer. Obstetrician James Young Simpson, who introduced chloroform and was the first obstetrician to utilize general anesthesia for labor and delivery, countered this protest with an ingenious argument. He pointed out that God Himself was the first to use general anesthesia: He removed a rib from Adam only after he was asleep! The resistance to ether and chloroform for surgical procedures soon ended, although, as discussed earlier, resistance to anesthesia during labor persists up to the present day.

At the fiftieth anniversary of Morton's fateful demonstration of ether, poet Weir Mitchell summed up the impact of that demonstration nicely:

> *Whatever triumphs still shall hold the mind,*
> *Whatever gift shall yet enrich mankind,*
> *Ah! here no hour shall strike through all the years,*
> *No hour as sweet, as when hope, doubt, and fears,*
> *'Mid deepening stillness, watched one eager brain,*
> *With Godlike will, decree the Death of Pain.*

11 THE SHADOWLANDS OF PAIN

"I am half sick of shadows,"
said the Lady of Shalott...

—Alfred, Lord Tennyson, "The Lady of Shalott"

I have treated some nightmarish pain problems in my career, including trigeminal neuralgia, disseminated prostate cancer, massive heart attacks, postherpetic neuralgia, belligerent kidney stones, and traumatic amputations. I've seen patients writhe in uncontrolled torment from ruptured spinal discs and fractured vertebrae. I've watched hundreds of people wince, limp, and vomit their way through life because of arthritis, diabetic neuropathy, or migraines. I've witnessed the agonies of childbirth countless times. But of all the pain-stricken patients I've treated over the past twenty years, the hardest to treat are those with no obvious disease at all. These patients live in the Shadowlands.

Consider Hank, a twenty-eight-year-old firefighter injured on the job. He wasn't hurt fighting a fire but instead fell victim to a freak accident at his station house. He had just made himself a cup of coffee and was leaning back to read the morning paper when his chair abruptly gave way. It was an old office chair with wheels and a spring-loaded back; the spring broke under Hank's weight and sent him sprawling to the floor. He fell hard on the concrete, spilling his hot coffee and causing a second-degree burn on the front of his right thigh. His coworkers immediately picked him up, dusted him off, and drove him to the nearest emergency room. Thus began Hank's sad saga of failed medical therapies and ceaseless litigation.

I first saw Hank two years after the accident. He had yet to return to work, and while his leg burns healed without a trace, he still complained bitterly of pain in his right thigh and lower back. He entered my office leaning hard on a cane, limping and moaning with every step. Not thirty years old, Hank's hunched posture, slow gait, and contorted face made him look old. A heavy black brace cloaked his lumbar spine and painkilling electrodes dotted his right thigh. Simply undressing and climbing onto my examination table took him many agonizing minutes.

In the years since his fall, Hank endured months of chiropractic manipulations and physical therapy to no avail. He was now enrolled in a pain management clinic, undergoing weekly injections of steroids and analgesics into his spine and legs. Every other afternoon he spent in an aquatherapy program, exercising in a large swimming pool to keep his back limber. He also consumed a staggering menagerie of drugs—morphine compounds, antidepressants, muscle relaxers, and sleep aids.

Hank's wife accompanied him to his visit carrying a mountainous assortment of MRI scans, myelographic X rays, electrical nerve studies, and physician reports. She also came armed with a thick, worn diary and took copious notes of everything I did and said during the hour I spent with them—"for our lawyers." They wanted to tape-record my examination as well, but I politely refused.

Examining Hank proved a laborious affair. He could scarcely

move without gasping in pain. I couldn't even touch his lower back without eliciting yelps so loud that they alarmed the patients outside in my waiting room. He refused to perform such elementary tasks as bending over, standing on his toes, or rotating his waist, saying that such maneuvers would "put me in bed for three days" (even though he had bent at the waist to remove his shoes and socks without protest). All the while, his wife scribbled furiously in her diary, occasionally glancing at her watch to see how long I took to perform each aspect of the examination.

Hank was a walking paradox. His six-foot frame fairly rippled with well-defined muscles and bulging veins, and he looked like a bodybuilder in training, despite years of professed inactivity. Either he possessed an exceptionally fine set of genes or was much more active than he cared to admit. He couldn't even walk the fifty-odd feet to his mailbox, or so he claimed, without having to rest for hours afterward. Nevertheless, his legs looked and felt like pillars of iron.

Hank's hands were filthy and covered with healed cuts and heavy calluses, another indication that he was lying about his level of activity. I pointedly asked him about the battered appearance of his hands and he replied that he had "an inherited skin condition" that made them look that way. His wife rolled her eyes in indignation as I queried him on this issue but said nothing.

Finally, I looked into Hank's eyes: he had large pupils, not the pinpoint dots I would have expected from a man almost marinating himself in morphine compounds. Something didn't fit here.

After my exam I instructed husband and wife to return to the relative comfort of my waiting area while I retired to an adjoining room to review Hank's records and X-ray films. All the facts pointed to the same conclusion: nothing was wrong with Hank, at least not physically. His spine studies and nerve testing looked normal. Two other spine surgeons and a neurologist had also evaluated Hank in the past, all of whom declined to get involved with the case because of an apparent absence of any real disease or injury. His current physician—a certified pain specialist—recently diagnosed Hank with "chronic pain syndrome" secondary to "work-related spinal disc trauma," although she never specified which discs were traumatized. His discs looked fine to me. In addition to sticking needles in him every week, his pain specialist also dispensed those invaluable slips of paper he needed to claim permanent disability status.

I gleaned a few other interesting facts from Hank's records. He currently received workers' compensation pay for his injuries; a separate disability insurance policy covered his mortgage while he was off work. Adding these two sources of income—and adjusting for tax benefits afforded to injured workers—Hank made more money injured than he earned while working full-time. In addition, he was suing the city and the manufacturer of the broken chair.

Insurance documents listed the cost of Hank's medical care at about a hundred thousand dollars...and counting. The insurance companies continued to spend about fifteen hundred dollars a week for his aquatherapy, spinal injections, and drugs, despite the lack of evidence that he had ever been seriously injured. And they continued to pay even though these therapies gave him no pause from his perceived sufferings.

I gathered together the records and films and summoned Hank and his spouse back to the privacy of my exam room. "I have nothing to offer you," I said as I returned the stack of materials. Hank's wife resumed her scribbling. "I see nothing wrong here."

"What am I supposed to do? They told me an operation is my only hope." Hank's voice was thick with anger.

"You don't need an operation," I replied. "That should be good news. Operations can be risky business."

They took the films and shuffled sullenly out of the door.

⮞

Medical science has no objective way to measure pain. A number of "quantitative" methods for evaluating pain have been devised, such as the Borg scale, which consists of asking patients to rate their pain on a scale of zero (no pain) to ten (the maximum pain they have ever personally experienced), and the visual scale, wherein a patient is shown a drawing of a pain "thermometer" and instructed to mark how high up the thermometer their own pain reaches. All of these scales share a common weak link: they measure only the patient's perception of pain, not the pain itself. There's no independent way of confirming that someone who claims to be in severe pain actually is. Why is this important? Because many pain therapies carry great risks and should not be used unless those applying them are reasonably confident that the pain is real.

Centuries ago philosopher Plato proposed a cave analogy to describe the physical world. Envision, mused Plato, people in a cave who face a blank wall. They are chained so that they cannot look behind them, where a roaring fire burns. As the people watch the wall, a deer walks behind them and they see the shadow of the deer on the wall cast by the light of the fire. They mistake the flickering image for a living thing; because the shadow mimics the true deer, Plato's people can make some valid observations based on the shadow alone—for example, the shadow deer, like the true deer, owns a head, four legs, and a tail. But without seeing the flesh-and-blood animal, they can never know the color of its fur. Because of their limited perception, Plato's cave people can know only an approximation of the deer, not the deer itself.

To Plato, everyday objects are like shadows on the cave's wall. We see a projection of things, not their true nature. That nature lies in an abstract world of absolute truth, a world that we can never see. C. S. Lewis put a religious spin on Plato's cave model, stating that the human body is nothing but the shadow cast by an immortal soul upon the world. We live in the Shadowlands, say Lewis and Plato, seeing only incomplete illusions and not absolute reality.

Pain physicians also must work in a sort of Shadowlands. It's a place where people seem to suffer greatly, but we don't know why. The Shadowlands harbor all of those patients who experience pain out of proportion to any apparent ailment or injury.

We cannot see, feel, smell, or touch pain felt by other people. We see only the shadow that pain casts upon their lives. We can feel our own pain, but the pain of others lies beyond our senses. In Plato's model, shadows tell us something but not everything: a mouse could throw a shadow as large as an elephant if the optics were just right, but a mouse is not an elephant. Minor illnesses and trivial injuries may likewise cast an exaggerated shadow on the lives of their victims. In Hank's case, one small fall from a chair seemed to ruin his life, even though his mild injuries had apparently healed. Hank lived in the Shadowlands. The shadow I saw in my office looked huge and monstrous, but was his pain itself that menacing?

The shadow of pain can look quite real, even when there's no pain behind it at all. In the dramatic opening scene of the film *Saving Private Ryan,* we see a hundred men cut to pieces by enemy gun fire. One image in particular—a soldier screaming in agony as a medic tries to suture the ragged stump of his freshly amputated arm—so disturbed me that I had dreams about it almost nightly for several weeks. But this man had no pain. He was an actor, and his stump, with its exposed nerves and pumping arteries, merely a Hollywood prop made of plastic. Nevertheless, I felt that actor's bogus pain to the core of my being and was shaken by it just as I would have been shaken by actual pain. This false shadow was so lifelike that I was terrified by it, like a child terrified by the shadow of a tree on his bedroom wall that he mistakes for a ghost.

In life, as in the movies, physicians and other health care providers run across actors who can create a convincing, albeit false, illusion of great pain. We call these people malingerers, people who can be proven to be lying about their pain. Why would people lie about pain? For three reasons: money, narcotics, and control.

In litigious societies, monetary awards in civil suits are often calculated according to "pain and suffering." Similarly, most cases of workers' compensation and permanent disability determinations involve chronic pain syndromes. In this context, pain becomes a tangible commodity that can be bought and sold in the marketplace, occasionally for exorbitant amounts of money. In a recent malpractice settlement, a jury awarded a man $7 million for complaints of chronic back pain after a failed disc operation. The man had no medical complications from his operation and still managed all of his daily activities; the money was awarded for his pain only. With sums like this at stake, the temptation to lie about pain can be great, even for people we would not otherwise consider evil or criminal. I call the use of pain to extract money the Reverse Inquisition.

During the original Inquisition, pain was used by authority

figures as a tool to extract something of value from victims: a confession, money, an oath of loyalty, the betrayal of a friend. But the situation has been turned on its head. Today people use pain as a tool to leverage something of value from authority figures, usually insurance companies or the government. Pain, once the instrument of the State against the Common Man, now becomes the Common Man's weapon against the State.

The desire for narcotic drugs can provide an equally strong temptation for malingering. Patients start out with a real malady, become addicted to pain pills, and then find they must continue to complain of pain in order to obtain their prescriptions. The physician becomes faced with a dilemma: Is this person really in pain or simply seeking pain medications for recreational use (or for resale on the street to other addicts)? When I was working in emergency rooms, I had a patient who was seen traumatizing his own bladder with a coat hanger so that he would urinate blood and convince us he had a kidney stone—just to receive a single shot of morphine and then vanish.

Finally, there is the issue of control, also called secondary gain. In this instance, pain isn't used to extract something of personal gain but as a tool to control others. Years ago when I treated many cases of facial pain, I was struck by the number of patients who first noticed their pain at difficult points in their marriages. One woman, for example, had the onset of pain when she discovered that her husband was having an affair. Her painful condition soon consumed so much of his time—taking her to physicians around the country, running to the pharmacy, calling off work to stay at home with her—that his illicit affair soon dissolved. Pain can also be used as a subtle form of blackmail, often against employers as a means of obtaining better jobs. A nurse, tired of lifting patients all day, may claim an occupational back injury and threaten to sue his employer unless he gets a better-paying teaching position in the nursing school that will be easier on his spine.

★

Shouldn't altruistic healers discount base economic, drug-seeking, or control motives on the part of patients and simply treat all pain at face value? Should healers be in the position of accusing their patients of lying?

There are no easy answers to these questions, but, unfortunately, issues such as litigation status and substance abuse can have such a great impact on the diagnosis and management of pain syndromes that they cannot be ignored. From a practical standpoint, it's difficult to treat people in the Shadowlands in the same way we treat patients with documented disease. For example, over 90 percent of nonlitigating patients enjoy a good outcome from spinal surgery; in patients involved in workers' compensation lawsuits at the time of their surgery, however, the success rate can be as low as 40 or 50 percent—about the same as being on a placebo. Thus, it becomes questionable whether a patient involved in a lawsuit can be ethically offered surgery at all, given the dismal outcomes. Many surgeons are of the opinion that litigating patients should still be offered surgery because their poor outcomes can't be real. The patients, these surgeons argue, are indeed better after surgery but won't say so for fear of hurting their chances in court. But if these patients are lying about their level of pain after surgery, maybe they were lying about it before their surgery, too. This is the danger of practicing medicine in the Shadowlands. We may hurt people without real diseases, using powerful weapons like surgery. In the case of spinal operations, a patient's legal status becomes a prognostic factor for outcome equal to such medical factors as diabetes or a bad heart.

Pain surgeons must be on their guard against patients solely looking for a "red badge of courage" to validate their claims of injury. In the Civil War novel by Stephen Crane, the "red badge of courage" was a war wound, proof positive that a soldier had endured combat. In pain medicine, the red badge of courage is an operative incision. Patients may seek out an operation not because they have real pain but because an operation legitimizes their complaints.

Some may find it hard to believe that a person would submit to an operation simply for financial gain, but young prostitutes risk their lives every night for twenty dollars. Addicts inject lethal substances into their bodies solely for a few minutes of amusement. After twenty years in clinical medicine, I've ceased to be amazed by what people will do to their own bodies (see the coat hanger story above).

━➤

Hank and his wife brought lots of films and records with them, but they didn't know that the most important bit of information about his case had been mailed to me several days before his office visit. It consisted of a thirty-minute videotape made in Florida about six weeks earlier. Hank and his wife had gone to Florida at the time, ostensibly to visit his brother.

The insurance company paying Hank's claim contracted a private investigator in the Fort Myers area to keep an eye on him during his stay there. The Hank on the videotape was not the Hank I saw in my office. Gone were the cane and stooped posture; gone were the grimacing and moaning. I watched as Florida

Hank drove a motorized ski device through the pounding surf, and then lifted and carried the dripping machine—weighing over a hundred pounds—onto the beach. Hank, it seemed, was a bona fide malingerer. He eventually landed in prison.

Still, I didn't accuse him of faking. I merely exercised my medical judgment by not offering him any surgery. Hank's case isn't a morality tale of good versus evil, but a stark example of the difficulties encountered when treating patients whose pain seems out of proportion to objective evidence of real disease, the Shawdowlands patients. Had I crippled him with an operation, I would have injured a perfectly healthy man for no reason. Thus, my suspicions about him were for his own good. Hank's chiropractor and pain specialist treated him in good faith—they were unaware of the video evidence I had received. Nevertheless, they consumed thousands of dollars of insurance money and exposed Hank to needless risk while treating his imaginary pain shadow.

Although Hank's case is illustrative, he's by no means typical. Needless to say, most chronic pain patients, including patients involved in legitimate litigation, are not malingerers. Even when patients have no identifiable source of discomfort, there's every reason to believe that *something* is going on. In many cases the disease is there; we just haven't found it.

In some patients the presence of severe pain is verified by objective pathology, like the presence of cancer, a fracture, or a large ruptured disc in the spine. In other instances patients have no clearly visible pathology but provide such a classic constellation of complaints that their diagnoses aren't in doubt. Trigeminal neuralgia and migraines are good examples of pain syndromes that can be reliably diagnosed by the patient's story alone. Sometimes, however, patients have no pathology and voice weird or atypical complaints, raising the specter of malingering.

But before rushing to judgment and suspecting patients of inflating or imagining their pains, we must remember that a number of well-recognized syndromes started out as "weird and atypical." In centuries past vascular headaches were thought to be manifestations of evil spirits. In our own century many women with chronic muscular discomfort were written off as hopeless whiners before we understood the entity now known as fibromyalgia. Some doubted that trigeminal neuralgia had an organic basis until Dandy discovered its cause at the base of the brain. The earliest victims of Lyme's arthritis also encountered skepticism about their vague and random symptoms before laboratory confirmation of their disease became available. Just because someone seems to be free of disease when imaged or tested with current technology does not mean that they are indeed healthy and malingering. Our current technology may simply be unable to detect the true source of their pain; future technology may change that situation.

Occasionally we already have the technology to diagnose a condition but fail to use it properly. Two months ago I treated a woman for chronic hip pain "of unknown etiology"; her spinal scans showed no disc disease and plain X rays of the hip were normal. A bone scan, on the other hand, revealed a hairline stress fracture in the head of the femur. An orthopedic surgeon pinned the hip and she was relieved of her pain within a few days. In this case she had real disease, although she almost ended up discarded into the Shadowlands.

Some neurophysiologists believe that chronic pain resides in the brain, not in the body. Although the original source of the pain may be outside the brain—a ruptured disc, a broken bone— this bodily pain can eventually activate a pain center in the brain, perhaps in the thalamus (the sensory clearinghouse deep within the cerebral hemispheres), and once activated it's never silent again. The activated pain center continues to transmit pain signals into the consciousness long after the bodily hurt has healed, a phenomenon analogous to that which occurs in hyperactive spinal nociceptive neurons during anesthesia dolorosa. Quite literally, the pain is "all in our heads." If these physiologists are correct, the answer to many chronic pain syndromes lies not in treating the body but in treating the brain, using thalamic lesioning and stimulators or by pumping narcotics directly into the head.

The most promising approach to pain originating in activated brain centers may lie in drugs that act preferentially within the brain to quiet misbehaving neurons, drugs like ziconotide produced by the Neurex Corporation and ABT-594, a substance extracted from the Ecuadorian tree frog by Abbott Laboratories. As our understanding of central brain pain improves, many pain patients who appear disease free today may later emerge from the shadows and be shown to have an organic brain ailment that can be treated successfully.

The Shadowlands also harbor another confounding diagnosis: psychiatric pain. About two thirds of psychiatric outpatients have some complaint of pain even though most have never had any physical illness or injury. Intractable atypical headache and abdominal pain are particularly common among patients suffering from severe psychiatric illness.

A failure to perceive or accept reality is a recurring theme among many psychiatric diagnoses. The schizophrenic hears voices that don't exist; the obsessive-compulsive checks her oven again and again, even though she turned it off herself only hours ago; the depressed Pulitzer Prize–winning author harbors delusional feelings of utter worthlessness; the paranoid thinks that the waitress is plotting against him; the agoraphobe believes that a local supermarket offers insurmountable dangers; and so on. Most mental illnesses, even those that don't cause frank psychosis, distort a person's perception of reality to a certain degree. In this context, the tendency of a psychiatric patient to convert trivial or nonexistent physical ailments into lifelong torments becomes understandable. The schizophrenic hears ghost voices and suffers ghost headaches. Menstrual cramps become a sign of lethal disease to the neurotic. Obsessives ruminate over ordinary toothaches and back pains.

Psychiatric patients are not malingerers—they believe they have pain. Indeed, they probably do have pain, even though they rarely respond to any conventional pain therapies. Every year I see at least one or two schizophrenic patients with headaches who are convinced that they suffer from tumors despite having perfectly normal brain scans. Their psychiatrists refer them to me hoping that I, as a brain surgeon, can convince them of their folly. I can't, of course, but I try. I display their scans alongside the scans of real brain tumors, carefully noting the differences and reassuring them in my most avuncular manner that there's nothing for them to worry about. They nod, go home, and promptly make preparations for their impending death from brain cancer.

Not surprisingly, their delusional headaches will not respond to anything we have to offer. Pain pills, nerve blocks, antiinflammatory medications, nothing will relieve their pain. Why? Because their pain, like their unshakable faith in fictional brain tumors, exists only in the Shadowlands of their minds. Pain pills are like negative scans—objects from the real world, objects that can never impact what they feel and believe. Their pain derives from their faulty interface with the outside world and that includes a distorted perception of their own bodies. It's a psychological pain, almost a kind of metaphysical pain, that does not answer to real-world entities like morphine or aspirin. The solution to this type of pain lies in the realm of psychiatry, not pain medicine.

The key to understanding pain in the Shadowlands may lie in rejecting the classic Cartesian view of pain entirely. Three hundred years ago mathematician and philosopher René Descartes formulated the "bell ringer" model of pain in which he portrayed pain as a purely quantitative phenomenon designed to alert us to physical injury. Descartes believed that there was a linear relationship between organic disease and pain, just as there is a linear relationship between how hard we pull the bell's ringer and how loud the bell rings.

The Cartesian model expresses in fancy language what we intuitively believe about pain: the bigger the injury, the bigger the hurt. Stubbing a toe won't hurt as much as having it cut off by the lawn mower; burning a finger won't hurt as much as burning the whole arm. Serious scientists know that what seems intuitive is not always correct, however, and the Cartesian model of pain is no exception. For example, in a famous study of war injuries conducted by Henry Beecher during World War II, soldiers with the most horrendous injuries often felt no pain, while soldiers with minor injuries sometimes had severe pain. Beecher found that Descartes's theory was all wrong: there is no linear relationship between injury and the perception of pain.

Descartes failed to take into account the human dimension of pain, a dimension that introduces a large degree of "nonlinearity" into the equation. The influence of psychological, social, religious, and economic issues can be so great that the magnitude of pain can become uncoupled from physical illness or injury altogether. Thus, the Shadowlands emerges. The Shadowlands is not an evil place. Instead, I see it as an uncharted frontier that may harbor the secrets to understanding human pain in all of its forms, Cartesian and otherwise.

As a physician, my job isn't to search out fraud or to play the role of insurance investigator. I don't police the Shadowlands for the good of society at large, but choose to treat individuals one at a time and in their best medical interests. Nevertheless, we as caregivers must respect the hazards that still lie there, and we cannot allow ourselves to become pawns in legal skirmishes or greedy participants in a chronic pain game, performing procedures we know are worthless simply in exchange for fees.

Some pain specialists avoid the Shadowlands entirely by refusing patients with psychiatric problems, ongoing litigations, or undocumented disease. Other caregivers simply give every patient anything he or she wants—endless spinal manipulations, weekly nerve blocks, addictive drugs, major operations, anything at all—enriching themselves in the process. I have taken a different road, treating any patient who seeks my help without exception, but not taking every complaint as gospel truth.

Like any neurosurgical office, mine sees an endless parade of accident victims and people seeking drugs. Half of my new patients have acquired attorneys by the time of their initial office visit, and I now spend almost as much time testifying about injuries as I do treating them. My stomach becomes twisted in knots every time I have to make a decision about whether to believe patients' complaints or suspect them of inflating their pain. I wish I could believe everything of my patients, but that's not good medicine.

Sometimes those of us caring for pain patients in the Shadowlands lose our way in the great darkness. But until we can turn toward the fire and see Plato's deer, observing every patient's pain in the flesh, we must continue to wander in pain's Shadowlands and do the very best we can.

12 THE AGONIES OF THE CRAB

I'm jus' pain covered in skin. I know what it is…

—the dying Mrs. Wilson,
in John Steinbeck's *The Grapes of Wrath*

Steinbeck never tells us what's wrong with Mrs. Wilson, the impoverished woman befriended by the Joads during their sojourn to California. But his readers should recognize her disease: cancer. After reading Steinbeck's powerful descriptions of Mrs. Wilson's torment, can we have any doubt about "what it is"?

During my nearly twenty years in clinical medicine, I have seen too many people who, like Mrs. Wilson, had been reduced by cancer to "jus' pain covered in skin." Willa Knoltz was one. I first met Willa several years ago at McKeesport Hospital when her oncologist requested my aid in controlling her escalating pain. Willa was a frail wisp of a woman in her midseventies. Her diminutive stature, fine facial features, and porcelain-smooth complexion made her look like an animated doll as she moved slowly and quietly about her room. Her meticulously coiffured hair showed that she had not yet received any toxic forms of chemotherapy. I took this as a bad sign—she was already in trouble with pain control and hadn't even started any curative therapy. I surmised that she must have advanced disease, too advanced to consider toxic chemotherapy at all. My conclusion proved correct.

Willa had been having left leg pain for several months. The pain began in a small way, as great pains often do. At first just a faint gnawing deep within her thigh, it quickly built to a crescendo of discomfort and now bubbled like molten lava from her bone, flowing upward into the hip joint and downward to the knee. Walking worsened the pain terribly, but it was there even when lying down. Within a month she had progressed from taking an occasional aspirin to gulping narcotics round-the-clock, yet the pain always remained a step ahead of the drugs.

There are many benign causes of hip and leg pain at Willa's age: spinal disc problems with pinched nerves, inadequate circulation, muscle cramping, arthritic hip disease, various forms of neuropathy. Her physician evaluated each of these diagnoses and, not surprisingly, found evidence to support all of them to some degree. Plain X rays showed Willa's hip was arthritic; an MRI of her spine identified two spinal discs that were deteriorating; vascular studies of her legs found that her circulation, although not terrible, wasn't in the best of shape either; and electrical evaluation of her nerves turned up some minor damage there as well. This left Willa and her doctor with too many answers and, at the same time, with no answers at all. They had identified many little diseases but not the big one capable of spawning such intense pain. A big disease was there all right but had yet to be discovered.

Seeking relief, Willa went to a vascular surgeon; he found that her circulation wasn't diseased enough to be responsible for severe pain. He patiently explained to her that vascular pain normally comes on after activity and since Willa's pain was there all the time, hers couldn't be vascular pain. Next she went to a spine surgeon who found nothing to offer, either. The discs were bad, he noted dispassionately, but weren't pressing on the nerves to her legs and so could not be causing any pain.

The better part of three months was quickly consumed in a vain search for the origin of her pain. During that time the problem worsened. As the thigh discomfort escalated, Willa began to descend into depression and she soon became overwhelmed with the fear that nothing was wrong, that she was merely falling apart from old age.

Finally, Willa's internist referred her to an orthopedic surgeon. The orthopedist quickly ordered a bone scan to assess the degree of inflammation in Willa's arthritic hip. To perform a bone scan, technicians first inject an intravenous radioactive substance that becomes concentrated in areas of the skeleton that are inflamed or are undergoing destruction and remodeling. The technicians then "photograph" the skeleton using film sensitive to radioactivity. Abnormal areas show up as "hot spots" on the film.

Ordinary X rays are static images that reveal bone structure only. Bone scanning, on the other hand, is a dynamic test that "sees" active processes like bone healing that may be invisible on X rays. Bone scanning can even uncover tiny fractures in otherwise normal-appearing bone. If the scan proved Willa's hip was "cold," the arthritic changes seen on the plain X rays were unlikely to be responsible for her pain. If the scan was "hot," Willa's hip was probably so badly inflamed that only a new hip joint would cure her.

Willa's hip was cold—but something unexpected turned up. The scan revealed hot spots in two ribs as well as in the lower shaft of her left femur, or thigh bone. When her internist received a copy of Willa's bone scan report, he knew immediately what these hot spots meant and his heart sank. Eight years earlier Willa had undergone a lumpectomy and radiation to treat a small cancerous mass detected in the right breast on routine mammography; this cancer, once thought gone forever, was back. Willa's problem wasn't old age but something worse: metastatic cancer.

Willa's internist hadn't suspected cancer earlier because so many years had passed since the successful breast surgery. Unfortunately, breast cancer can be a strange malady, lying dormant for decades before resurfacing with a vengeance. A needle aspirate of Willa's femur confirmed the presence of metastatic breast cancer. By the time I saw her, no bone scans or needle biopsies were needed to make the diagnosis of metastatic disease. Only one thing can produce that much misery on someone's face—I saw her cancer staring back at me through her weary eyes.

Further outpatient testing found cancerous spots in Willa's liver and lungs, too; saving her life quickly became a lost cause. Her doctors now turned their attention to a task no less daunting: easing her relentless suffering.

I vividly recall a lecture given by Rabbi Harold Kushner to a national gathering of neurosurgeons a number of years ago. Kushner, a noted expert on dying and the author of *When Bad Things Happen to Good People,* stressed that cancer patients aren't so much afraid of death as they are terrified of the process of dying. Kushner felt that dying with cancer had become synonymous with dying in great pain. Unfortunately, this belief remains true even today. Three of four cancer patients will die in poorly controlled pain, and the percentage climbs higher still for those succumbing to malignancies with a talent for invading bones and nerves, including cancers of the breast, prostate, rectum, pancreas, and cervix. Not surprisingly, the treatment of pain quickly dominates the medical, social, and psychological care of the typical end-stage patient.

Ironically, although pain is a common problem in advanced cancers, malignancy rarely causes pain as an initial symptom. In their earliest stages, for example, tumors of the breast, lung, skin, and prostate may be entirely painless. In fact, a "painless lump" may be a more ominous discovery than an exquisitely painful one, since the latter is more likely to be an abscess or another benign process. Unless they cause palpable swellings or visible bleeding, most cancers progress silently until they disseminate throughout the body.

This lack of early pain seems a rather curious and paradoxical thing, given pain's supposed role as a warning bell. What good is a warning bell that sounds only after the danger proves irreversible? Isn't pain that alerts someone to end-stage cancer like a smoke detector that goes off after the house has been reduced to cinders?

But when viewed in its proper biological context, the lack of pain in the first stages of cancer makes merciful sense. Humankind has been dying of cancer for a thousand centuries but has only been able to treat it with any success for the past few decades. Two hundred years ago, in the era before mammography and radiotherapy, a breast tumor no bigger than a mosquito's head already doomed its host to death. In the natural world—a world devoid of artificial therapies—cancer never has a "curable" stage. Warning signs of cancer are useless in natural populations, given the unstoppable nature of the disease. We do get pain from cancer, of course, but only in its more terminal phases.

Cancer's procrastination in creating pain is a good thing,

given the long life span of many tumors. We tend to think of cancer as a rapid process; in fact, it can progress quite slowly, particularly in its infancy. Many years often pass before the first mutant tumor cells proliferate to a size capable of causing clinical symptoms. That final explosive growth phase we know as "cancer" is merely an endgame in the long (and largely silent) struggle between parasite and host.

This is the merciful side of cancer. By causing us no pain during its formative years, cancer lets us live in ignorant bliss as it slowly overwhelms our bodies. If cancer didn't leave us alone for the bulk of its life span, it would prove an even nastier adversary. Consider the breast cancer patient of two hundred years ago. Had her pain started when the tumor was vanishingly small, she would have had to endure the pain helplessly for ten, maybe even twenty years before the cancer finally claimed her life. Instead, the disease grows stealthily until it makes its way to the bone. True, at that point she will know great pain for months before she dies, but that's a few months of symptoms from a disease spanning many years. This may be the best we can hope for in a biological world notoriously bereft of mercy. In a sense, cancer proves a much kinder illness than "benign" entities like osteoarthritis or trigeminal neuralgia, illnesses that torture for years without killing.

And when cancer decides to claim us, it can do so with great speed. Metastatic cancer is a matador that makes its victims dance briefly before the veronica before rapidly putting the sword to their hearts. Like our belief that cancer is curable, the belief that cancer is a lingering illness is a modern and artificial one, yet another illusion created by our advanced technologies. Cancer lingers because of our great efforts to stave it off. Left alone, it kills with stunning velocity. Prior to the advent of modern medical interventions, suffering from metastatic disease was intense but brief. True, our technology has given us better tools to deal with cancer pain, but this technology also works against the greatest of all natural painkillers: a swift death.

If pain has no biological role in cancer's early stages, then it certainly serves no purpose in its later stages. So why have cancer pain at all? Why can't we just dwindle away in anesthetic oblivion as cancer consumes us, drifting off to sleep when our tumor burden finally grows too large to support life? Why are we so keenly aware of a disease from which there is no natural escape? To understand this enigma, we must understand the nature of cancer pain.

Cancer pain arises not from the lumps of tumor themselves, but from the mechanical disruptions they cause throughout the body. The skeleton, as the body's supporting framework, is at particular risk for such disruptions. Consequently, bone metastases produce the lion's share of cancer's miseries.

In Willa's case, the metastatic tumor in her femur caused a structural flaw in the bone similar to that caused by a recent or poorly healed leg fracture. As soft tumor grew within the long shaft of her femur, it slowly replaced the bone's harder elements, causing a progressive weakening of the thigh, like soft rust compromising a steel beam. The skeleton possesses a thin outer wrapping of tissue called periosteum (meaning "around the bone"), which is exquisitely sensitive to abnormal bending or distortion of the underlying bone. Stretching or buckling of the periosteum, even to the tiniest degree, will cause intense pain. The periosteum of the tibia, or shinbone, lies just beneath the skin; those wishing to assess the sensitivity of their periosteum need only strike their shins firmly against a coffee table. Most people, I suspect, will take me at my word and forego this experiment.

Periosteal pain provides an essential protective function. It forces us to rest broken limbs until the bone knits and becomes solid once more. It also tells us when the weights we lift or the acrobatics we attempt exceed the design limits of our skeletons. Periosteum thus prevents broken bones and helps heal them if they do break.

Needless to say, Willa's leg would never solidify properly because of the presence of cancer, but her periosteum doesn't know that. It's simply warning her of the impending collapse of her thigh bone without rendering any judgments as to whether that warning will prove useful or not in the long run. Thus, we see why end-stage cancers cause pain, even when that pain makes no prophylactic sense. By causing structural flaws in bones and other pain-sensitive organs, cancer triggers protective pain reflexes that evolved to maximize the healing of reversible processes. There is no intrinsic difference between benign and malignant pain—they are mechanistically one and the same. A deformed leg bone hurts, whether that deformity is caused by an irreversible cancer or by a reversible fracture resulting from a tumble off a horse. In the case of benign pain, the underlying pathologic process will resolve and the pain will eventually subside. In the case of malignant pain, on the other hand, the underlying process cannot resolve (at least not without medical intervention) and the pain can never subside. Willa's pain told her to rest her leg, even though rest alone could never make it heal.

Tumor masses wreak havoc in a number of other ways. Vertebrae weakened by cancerous invasion can collapse, crushing spinal nerves in the process. The muscles of the back then go into endless crippling spasms as they try to form a natural splint around the wobbly spine and prevent further nerve damage. Masses within the colon cause intestinal obstruction and cramping discomfort. Masses in the pancreas smash or invade the rich plexus of nerves in the posterior abdomen, causing severe pain radiating into the back and chest.

Even when it causes no structural weakness, a cancerous lump within bone can expand, pressing directly against the periosteum and causing localized pain and tenderness. Tumors within the brain exert pressure on the skull and its sensitive inner lining, yielding blinding headache. In all of these scenarios, the identical pain can be caused by benign reversible diseases—noncancerous cysts, infections, trauma, aneurysms, blood clots, and so on. For these benign diseases, pain serves as an essential component of the healing process by altering our behaviors in ways that maximize good functional outcome. To evolve free of the risk of cancer pain, we would have had to evolve without any of the pain-aversive behaviors essential to our survival. For Willa to be oblivious to her disease, she would need congenitally anesthetic thigh bones—not a safe design feature for an active biped.

From the Darwinian point of view, cancer is an unimportant disease. Since it preferentially afflicts animals beyond their childbearing years, cancer poses no threat to animals (or humans) in the wild, since natural populations experience death in other ways long before they are old enough for cancer to be a concern. We feel the sting of advanced prostate cancer because we are fortunate enough to live into our seventh decade and beyond, a feat rarely achieved even a hundred years ago. During the evolution of the nervous system, we developed pain to help us heal reversible insults: cracked vertebrae, pinched nerves, temporarily blocked colons, broken legs. To our great sorrow, this same pain also works against us when irreversible diseases like cancer strike; consequently, death becomes a painful affair. We die with all of our pain alarms impotently sounding.

It has been said that we are all born in another's pain and destined to die in our own. Unfortunately, the design of our nervous system makes this so. Our pain pathways scream out against anything that threatens us, and since we must all face a lethal threat eventually, we all face terminal pain no matter what disease ultimately claims us. The same periosteal sensitivity that protects the gazelle's frail leg as it dashes across the Serengeti will also torture the poor creature when the leg is rended by a lion's jaws. The same periosteal sensitivity that guarded Willa's thigh from injury as she danced at her wedding now seared a hole in her consciousness as she approached the twilight of her life.

I sensed that Willa was now caught in the cancerous whirlpool of suffering and was about to be sucked down. Unless we could quickly break the self-perpetuating cycle of pain, hopelessness, and despair, we might not be able to salvage a dignified death.

The ultimate goal of medicine is not, contrary to popular belief, achieving human immortality. Rather, our goal should be a world in which people live free of pain for ninety-nine years and then die peacefully in their sleep. The true business of a physician is not saving lives but easing pain. In the final analysis, none of our lives can really be saved, although we all crave a comfortable death.

A comfortable death was all that modern medicine had left to offer Willa. Unfortunately, there is no standard recipe for providing such a death. Comfortable deaths can't be prescribed like drugs or performed like operations. They have to be laboriously crafted and often the end result is still not entirely satisfactory.

For billions of years life has existed on this hostile planet for a single reason: living things don't take dying lightly. They don't go silently into that good night but prefer to exit kicking and screaming from life's stage. The human body has been built to survive; wrestling it quietly into the grave is no simple matter. Factor in the problems posed by human ethics and the desire to preserve some "quality of life" along with adequate pain control, and the difficulties faced by end-of-life caregivers become exponentially greater. Much has been written lately about the reluctance of physicians to provide the dying with adequate pain control. While it is true that we fail many patients, as Rabbi Kushner pointed out, it's also true that simultaneously providing a dying person with both pain control and a good quality of life is not easy. This is because strong pain requires strong medicine, and strong medicine always comes at a price.

Willa's cancer quickly spread to her spine and pelvis; although her mind came to accept the inevitability of her death, the diseased portions of her body still cried out with all their might to be rescued from the cancer that gripped them. Like passengers on a sinking ship, her mottled bones refused to accept that their craft was doomed and that they would eventually follow.

I tried first to rearrange her medications. In the early 1990s the World Health Organization formulated the "three-step analgesic ladder" for the medical management of cancer pain. The first rung consists of non-narcotic medications, including over-the-counter drugs like aspirin and acetaminophen and prescription anti-inflammatory agents like indomethacin. The second rung adds a mild narcotic (codeine, hydrocodone) to the first rung, and the third rung adds a potent narcotic (morphine, hydromorphone, fentanyl) to the first two rungs.

Willa was receiving a potent narcotic when I first met her, but she was not on any anti-inflammatory drugs. Her physicians had jumped directly to the third rung; moreover, the dosage of narcotic was too low. I switched her to a higher oral dose of long-acting morphine compound given twice daily and added a milder narcotic given every three hours together with indomethacin and some corticosteroids. We were able to get her out of the hospital and back to her normal life for about six weeks on this regimen before the pain began to escalate again. I raised the morphine dose every third day for another three or four weeks until I reached a dose of over half a gram of morphine a day—enough to kill a normal person. Willa, however, had been on morphine for almost three months by that time and had become resistant to the lethal properties of the drug. Just as longtime alcoholics can drink amounts of liquor that would kill a nondrinker, end-stage cancer patients can safely consume quantities of morphine deadly even to the hardened street addict. While morphine resistance makes the drug safer to use, it also reduces its efficacy and forces physicians to employ higher and higher doses.

Unfortunately, Willa didn't develop resistance to the sedation and the constipation produced by high-dose morphine. Heroin and other narcotics were first marketed as antidiarrheals because of their inhibitory effect on the colon; Willa had to be hospitalized twice just to have bowel movements. Even worse, she found herself dozing off in midsentence and could no longer be trusted to drive an automobile or to stand on a stool to water her beloved houseplants. The drugs strained her budget almost as badly as they strained her bowels. Although pain medications aren't particularly expensive, the huge number of pills she required on a daily basis was becoming a financial burden. One pack of cigarettes costs only a few dollars, but to the smoker who needs three packs every day, the cost soon mounts. The same is true of pain pills.

While I adjusted her narcotics, the radiotherapists attacked the cancerous sites of Willa's skeleton with their high voltage X rays, and the oncologists started her on tamoxifen, a nontoxic drug that inhibits breast cancer growth. Four months after the completion of radiotherapy, her bone tumors started to abate. New bone replaced the shrinking tumors and provided greater stability to her femur and spine. The pain eased, allowing reductions of her staggering drug regimen. This hiatus lasted a blissful year before the pain returned again.

The word *cancer* means "crab" and was given to the disease because of its tenacity, a singular ability to cling to its victim like a crab's claws clinging to its prey. The crab soon held Willa in a death grip. Radiotherapy is a good trick but can only be used once. Willa came back into the hospital late one night writhing in pain, accompanied by her tearful daughter. When I entered the room, Willa grabbed me by the lapels of my coat and said, "God help me," with the fierce desperation of someone being disemboweled before my eyes. The sight of her suffering made me nauseated, and I had to leave the room to collect myself.

I raised her oral dose of morphine, but that did nothing. She was at the point where she could barely take anything by mouth, and I was forced to start a continuous infusion of intravenous morphine. I took her to a point of lethargy with the infusion and still she moaned throughout the night. The following day I inserted a catheter into her lumbar spine and began injecting morphine directly into the spinal fluid in the hopes that the higher brain concentrations of narcotic would buy some time. If that worked, I could install a permanent morphine pump directly into her spine. The pump, which is completely beneath the skin and refilled weekly using a long hypodermic needle, might buy her another month or two of normal life. Maybe the cancer would take her by then. I found myself cheering the cancer on, hoping it would hurry up and finish the job. This sounds terrible coming from a physician, but it wasn't the first time that I prayed for a patient to die quickly. Willa's cancer refused to cooperate. Although the bone metastases became active again, the life-threatening growths in her liver and lungs languished. The tamoxifen was doing its job well. Although not really a curative chemotherapy, tamoxifen can be very effective in delaying death.

The spinal morphine infusion began and still she moaned. Her family and friends fidgeted uncomfortably in their chairs as she snored in her drugged slumber or cried out incoherently in a spasm of pain. In desperation, I replaced the spinal morphine infusion with marcaine, a local anesthetic, and gave her a complete spinal block; the moaning stopped. Since the bulk of her pain came from her back and legs, by rendering her lower body numb with a spinal anesthetic, I had instantly and totally relieved her pain. I lowered the dosage of narcotics, and within two days she was sitting up and chatting with her visitors. She was a new woman and I was hailed a hero. Those among us who had contemplated withdrawing her tamoxifen and steroids and allowing her tumor to overwhelm her now felt guilty as we saw the old Willa resurface like a modern Lazarus.

But I knew this was a Faustian bargain. In addition to being numb in her legs, she was also temporarily paralyzed from the waist down and unable to control her bowel and bladder. She couldn't live out her life under a spinal anesthetic; I feared I had done something terrible. For a few days she was completely without pain—the first time she had felt no pain in over a year and a half. That couldn't last, and soon she would be plunged back into a fog of suffering and drug-induced delirium. I was like a jailer taking a prisoner out to see the sun and smell the fresh air for a brief time before tossing her back into a rank dungeon forever. Better to have never brought her out at all. Still, it's hard to watch people suffer and do nothing. I now felt I was treating everyone's agony—hers, her family's, her friends'...even my own.

The most frequent complaint against physicians managing terminal pain is that they are too stingy with narcotics. The common wisdom states that we are so afraid of addiction and abuse that we don't give patients what they need. Although this is partly true, the idea that narcotics are the answer to all of our pain problems is false. There is no way narcotics can provide what the public demands: a pain-free but lucid death. The doses required to achieve freedom from pain are going to cause severe mental aberrations in most patients. Furthermore, narcotics are like retirement funds. Both have finite limits and their use must be calibrated according to the length of time they are needed. Like a spendthrift retiree who wastes his money long before he dies and winds up a pauper, the physician who is too liberal with narcotics early in the treatment of cancer pain may be surprised when death doesn't come quickly enough and the narcotic account runs dry. This was my mistake with Willa. Her liver metastases convinced me that she couldn't live another six months, and here she was pushing two years. I should have realized that a cancer that took years to metastasize may take years to kill. I hadn't bargained on the twin miracles of radiotherapy and tamoxifen. She now happily did needlepoint with her elbows propped up on anesthetic legs and looked to me to make this implausible situation permanent. But I had spent my ammunition, my guns were empty, and the enemy was still not slain.

⤜

I called in a friend of mine experienced with a procedure known as percutaneous cordotomy. I wasn't sure if Willa would benefit from cordotomy, but it was worth a try at this point. Pain sensations travel in the front of the spinal cord. Motor pathways travel in separate nerve bundles lying in the lateral aspect of the spinal cord and touch sensations lie to the rear of the cord. If we consider the spinal cord analogous to the torso, the pain pathways would reside in the abdomen, the motor pathways in the flanks, and the touch pathways in the back.

Pain from the lower body, particularly pain in the legs, can be ameliorated for up to a year by destroying the front half of the spinal cord either by cutting it under direct vision with a tiny knife or by burning it indirectly with a heated needle placed through the skin and into the cord under X-ray guidance. My friend was an expert in the needle version of this procedure. Done properly, the cordotomy renders the legs insensitive to pain while preserving normal touch and motor functions.

Cordotomy (from *tomos*, Greek for "to cut") has been around for decades. It was among the first modern major pain operations ever devised. On a personal note, one of my earliest recollections of television was a *Ben Casey* episode from the 1960s in which Casey, a neurosurgeon, was called upon to perform a cordotomy on a man screaming with cancer pain. I recall the happy man crying and hugging Casey after the successful operation. That image stuck with me forever. Even at that young age—I couldn't have been more than eight or nine years old—I realized that this was the greatest gift one person can give to another, the gift of relief, of comfort. Thirty years later and I now hoped my friend could give Willa that gift once and for all.

To do the operation, we had to let Willa's spinal block wear off. Since the biggest risk of cordotomy is the accidental destruction of motor pathways and resultant leg paralysis, we needed Willa awake and moving her legs to command. By having her wiggle her toes while we injured her spinal cord, we could be reasonably sure that the needle was in the right place. The spinal cord is no larger than the index finger; needle placement in cordotomy must be done to millimeter precision. Any hint of weakness in her legs and the procedure would have to be aborted. (Willa said she didn't care if she became paralyzed and would opt to continue even if paralysis occurred—an indication of the magnitude of her pain.)

As the spinal anesthetic wore off, Willa felt her leg being plunged once more into the boiling cauldron. She winced and gritted her teeth as we positioned the needle carefully and used the fluoroscope to verify its position among her tiny neck bones. Once certain of the correct position, we hooked the electrical generator to the needle and commenced burning the precious spinal cord. Within minutes we heard a tiny voice pipe up cheerily from beneath the green operating room drapes.

"It's gone. The pain. It's gone." Willa began to cry. I flashed back to three decades earlier, to that long-defunct television show. Sometimes life, like TV, has a happy ending.

For some strange reason, cordotomy typically relieves pain only in the legs, not pain in the back or torso, so Willa still suffered from pain in her vertebrae and ribs. This pain she could bear, however. The terrible pain that started it all, the pain in the left leg, would never return.

Like all destructive procedures, cordotomy carries the risk of delayed denervation pain, a burning discomfort that begins one or two years after the operation. For that reason, cordotomy can't be used when the patient is expected to live many years. Thus, it can't be used for benign leg pain caused by ruptured discs, vascular disease, diabetic neuropathy, or arthritic knees unless the patient has a concurrent terminal illness.

Willa's life fleshed out once again and for a short period she was no longer pain covered in skin. I feared that it was only a matter of time, though, before the other bone tumors became a problem. Before my fears materialized, fate intervened. Four months after her cordotomy, while shopping in a local supermarket, Willa gasped, clutched her chest, and collapsed to the floor. An hour later she was dead of a massive embolus to her lungs. Not the most peaceful of deaths to be sure, but, given the alternative, it would do. When I received the news of her sudden exodus, I felt genuinely happy for her. Good for you, Willa. You made it. You died standing with a bag of tangerines in your hand—when you could easily have died alone, confused, and tethered to my catheters.

Whenever we feel sorrow over a person's death, we should remember that all of us must cross the river Styx one day. We are only brief snapshots in the photo album of life on earth. As a physician, I have sworn an oath to make the journey as smooth as possible for my patients. But the crab is a difficult foe and its agonies cannot be fully mastered, at least not yet. New forms of narcotics and more precise pain surgeries may one day change this. For the present, however, the marriage of pain and death that was forged at the dawn of animal life remains a difficult union to break.

13   TO TREAT THE IMAGINATION

*The moral atmosphere surrounding the patient can
have a strong influence on the course of the disease.
It is not the curse or blessing that works, but the idea.
The imagination produces the effect.*

—Paracelsus (1493–1541)

Jack had severe low back pain. A body-and-fender man, he lifted heavy pieces of metal all day long and was taking pain pills by the dozens just to stay employed. He was addicted to codeine by the time I first saw him. I gave him an extended rest from work, prescribed physical therapy, and over three months managed to wean him off narcotics. But I couldn't get rid of all his pain. I experimented with a half dozen types of anti-inflammatory agents, three muscle relaxants, a transepidermal nerve stimulator (TENS), as well as two epidural steroid injections and some spinal joint blocks, but Jack's suffering smoldered away unchecked.

But one day Jack came into my office with a broad smile, claiming to be free of pain at last. "What," I asked, "brought about this abrupt miracle?" Jack unbuttoned his plaid shirt and displayed his cure: a back brace fitted with wafer-thin magnets. He had seen it advertised on television and had almost twisted an ankle running to the phone to order it. The device also came equipped with hard metal studs that were supposed to stimulate "acupuncture points" on the back and abdomen. "It makes you happy?" I asked. Jack nodded enthusiastically.

"Then," I replied with all sincerity, "it makes me happy, too."

Jack's story seems rather plain when compared to the more complex cases I have discussed previously. In a brief few months, however, Jack ran the gamut of available pain therapies, ranging from the hypermodern to the very ancient, before finally seeking refuge in a therapy that worked not on his body but on his imagination. Jack's case serves as the generic model for many common pain management problems.

We currently have three broad ways of treating any chronic pain: (1) eliminate the underlying cause; (2) treat the pain itself; or (3) alter the psychological perception of pain. This triad of strategies works best when used in that sequence: treat the cause first, the pain second, the psyche third.

The first strategy—attacking the cause of pain—achieves the best results by far; much of our modern success in pain management comes from a deepening understanding of disease and not from a better comprehension of pain itself. Better pain control comes from better disease control. The root cause of pain should always be addressed first, when possible.

Unfortunately, this is often *not* possible. Many patients suffer from incurable or untreatable illnesses. Jack's pain came from arthritic deterioration of his spinal joints, for which there is no long-term cure. Some patients fail to respond to maximal therapy even for normally curable problems. For example, about 10 percent of patients with sciatica will not obtain relief from disc surgery. In these instances, we must direct our long-term therapy at the pain itself. This can be done in one of three ways: narcotics, pain-masking devices, or ablative surgery. We've already seen several forms of ablative therapy—cordotomy for cancer pain, DREZ lesioning for brachial plexus avulsion, glycerol injection for trigeminal neuralgia. Since no ablative therapies exist for benign back pain, narcotics became Jack's first line of therapy. His internist prescribed them liberally before finally sending him to a specialist.

I use "narcotics" here in a colloquial sense to mean pain-killing prescription medications. The word *narcotic* derives from the Greek word for "stupor"; in earlier times, a narcotic was any drug that induced sleep. The story of painkilling narcotics dates back thousands of years to the first cultivation of a simple plant, the *Papaver somniferum*. This colorful flower, indigenous to Asia Minor, has been cultivated worldwide since ancient times; China, Turkey, India, and Egypt are now the dominant suppliers. The *Papaver* flower has a more common name: the poppy.

Unripe poppy seeds contain a milky juice that the Greeks named opium. The Greeks also contributed two other words to the lexicon of narcotics: *codeine,* from the word for the flower head itself, and *morphine,* named after Morpheus, the God of Dreams. When air-dried, poppy juice reduces to a brown paste that can be further processed into pure powdered opium. The Dutch called this paste *doop,* which later gave rise to the slang term *dope.* Raw opium powder contains almost two dozen active drugs known as opium alkaloids, a pair of which remain in common clinical use today: codeine and morphine.

Humankind has exploited the poppy for both recreational and medicinal purposes since prehistoric times. The first undisputed written reference to poppy juice (by Greek healer

Theophrastus) appeared in the third century before Christ. In the Middle Ages Arabian traders distributed processed opium throughout Asia, where it was used primarily to control dysentery. Opium then spread to Europe in the mid–sixteenth century, where physicians there began to take note of its painkilling properties. Paracelsus, the medieval physician who stumbled upon the sleep-inducing properties of ether, dissolved opium paste in alcohol and administered it to pain patients. He called this tincture *laudanum*—meaning "praiseworthy"—a name familiar to fans of Victorian literature.

In the nineteenth century a German pharmacist named Serturner succeeded in extracting pure morphine from raw opium powder, almost killing himself in the process. Other scientists purified additional opiate alkaloids, including codeine, shortly thereafter. With codeine and morphine commercially available, physicians could prescribe precise doses of painkillers instead of relying on haphazard preparations of poppy syrup. The industrial age of narcotics had begun.

Addiction and tolerance remain major stumbling blocks to the long-term use of opiates in chronic pain patients like Jack. While opiates provide excellent relief for acute benign pains (like the pain of surgery, bone fractures, bruises, and lacerations) and for malignant pain (which is often limited by a truncated life span), their application to protracted nonlethal maladies like arthritis, trigeminal neuralgia, fibromyalgia, and phantom pain remains problematic at best. Patients may respond initially to opiates, but soon require larger and larger doses to maintain their effect over time. Eventually the effective painkilling dose becomes too large to be sustained safely. Jack was taking sixteen codeine tablets a day when I first saw him, and their effect had largely dissipated.

With time any patient may develop a resistance to the pain-killing action of opiates, a phenomenon known as opiate tolerance. In order to achieve the same degree of relief, the patient must consume more and more of the drug. This is a problem distinct from addiction (also called dependence). The person dependent on opiates has a physical or mental craving for them and may become ill without them. The tolerant person, on the other hand, no longer obtains any benefit from the drugs and may stop taking them with little difficulty.

Because opiates work so well initially, patients often demand them. After they feel the immediate benefit of opiate drugs, they demand more. A prudent physician, aware of the Faustian bargain that chronic pain sufferers make with narcotics once they begin taking them, is understandably reluctant to dispense narcotics for chronic pain patients. This fear of narcotics isn't modern—healers in the second and third centuries warned of the addictive dangers of using poppy syrup for prolonged illnesses. Nevertheless, their hesitance to use opiates has created a false image of modern doctors as cruel and insensitive to pain, when nothing could be further from the truth. Physicians know that narcotics can often worsen a pain problem in the long run, not improve it. As a matter of fact, in many patients opiate use becomes their dominant problem, superceding the original pain problem over time. Long after the original injury heals, opiate addiction makes the patient feel as if something is still wrong. In Jack's case, weaning him off codeine actually lessened his pain in the long run.

How morphine and other opiate alkaloids work to reduce pain remained a mystery until the 1960s and 1970s, when scientists discovered naturally occurring brain proteins called opioids, or opium-like, to distinguish them from the plant opiates isolated from poppy juice. In pain medicine the most important of these opioids are the endorphins and enkephalins, which act like natural morphine.

Opioid hormones bind to specific opioid receptors in the brain and spinal cord. Opiate alkaloids (like morphine) and synthetic opiates (like fentanyl) mimic our natural endorphins and enkephalins and bind to the same opioid receptors within the nervous system. In fact, morphine and its synthetic cousins bind more avidly to these receptors than the natural substances themselves. In other words, artificial endorphins fit the locks of our body's painkilling doorways even better than the body's own endorphins. That's why we get greater relief (and a bigger rush) from morphine than we can from our own hormones.

There are two interesting evolutionary aspects to the opium story: (1) why do we have endogenous morphines floating in our brains in the first place, and (2) why would the sap of an Asian flower seed be so much better at relieving pain than our own bodies? The reason for the existence of endogenous morphines should be obvious. As we have seen, pain can be quite useful, in that it keeps us from walking on a broken leg and allows the bone to heal more quickly. At certain times, though, pain becomes counterproductive to survival. If a leg is shattered by an attacking grizzly bear, resting that leg will only facilitate our consumption by a hungry carnivore. Broken leg or not, we must run to live. In times of acute crises, endorphins and enkephalins mask pain for several hours, allowing us time to save ourselves or others despite massive injury.

Why the poppy makes such wonderful juice is also no mystery. Thanks to opium, the poppy has become the single most successful flower on the face of this earth. The poppy tempts us with its juice for its own survival. Stop and consider why such things as beautiful flowers and succulent fruits exist at all. The orchid doesn't put on a show for its own amusement and the pear tree doesn't cloak its seeds in tasty flesh because it has nothing better to do with its energies. Plants do these things to tempt animals, thereby enslaving more mobile creatures to do their bidding.

➤

After narcotics failed, the next thing we tried with Jack was the TENS unit, a pain-masking device. The use of pain-masking devices originated in the gate control theory of pain proposed by Melzack and Wall in 1965. The gate control theory postulates that pain sensations can be blocked by other sensations like touch or pressure. Touch and pressure travel along speedier pathways than pain sensations use, and they reach the spinal cord a fraction of a millisecond earlier. Once there, touch and pressure signals slam the gates shut behind them, excluding the more sluggish pain signals. The touch/pressure sensations then saturate the spinal cord's phone lines to the brain. In this way, a benign sensation can be used to mask an unpleasant sensation.

We have all used gate control pain masking at some time in our lives. If we accidentally scald one hand, we immediately grab it with the other and begin rubbing vigorously. Likewise, if we stub a toe or bang a shin on a table leg, we reflexively grab the damaged area and rub or apply pressure. Rubbing the feet of a patient with diabetic neuropathy or the leg of a patient with intractable sciatica will also help with their pain, but massaging a hurting area twenty-four hours a day is, needless to say, somewhat impractical for the average chronic pain patient. To exploit gate control masking in these patients, pain specialists employ devices that mimic cutaneous rubbing by electrically stimulating touch fibers in the skin (with TENS units) or nerve fibers within the spinal cord itself (using surgically implanted epidural stimulators). Both TENS units and epidural stimulators apply a gentle electric shock, either to the skin or the back of the spinal cord, via an array of electrodes. TENS electrodes are simply pasted to the skin, while epidural electrodes must be inserted by a neurosurgeon. Obviously, the TENS is cheaper, safer, and easier to use, but also much less effective. Both methods have modest benefits in properly selected patients.

The Melzack and Wall theory of pain represented a significant development in our basic understanding of pain to be sure, but I disagree with those authors who would rank it on a par with relativity theory or the discovery of the DNA double helix. The use of electricity to ease pain dates back to Roman times, when physicians stunned headache and gout victims with torpedo eels and electric skate fish; the idea that people could be shocked into ignoring their pain hardly originated with Melzack and Wall. Over the years I've become disenchanted by the long-term results produced by currently available pain-masking devices. Nevertheless, as we enter a new millennium and an era of exponentially expanding technologies, the gate control approach may yet change the face of pain management.

⤝

The last resort of pain control strategies—altering the perception of pain—remains the most mysterious. The human mind is the most important and least understood arena of modern pain management. We all suffer from the same diseases and injuries, but we don't perceive them in the same way. Although Jack wore his magnets around his waist, they probably did most of their healing within the confines of his skull.

The question for pain therapists becomes: How do we turn people who perceive their pain as a problem into people who don't? People have differing abilities to tolerate pain. Dancers and athletes exhibit a higher tolerance for physical pain compared to more sedentary subjects. Furthermore, a person's pain tolerance is not fixed in stone; we can be taught a higher tolerance of pain. Ancient Spartans strived diligently to manufacture soldiers who "laughed" at pain and deprivation; modern militaries do likewise. As a college student I couldn't get up for an eight o'clock class, but by the end of my surgical training I could work for forty-eight hours straight without wincing. Years of sleep deprivation hardened me and allowed me to ignore the weariness and suffering it causes. Can we use some form of pain "hardening" to treat chronic illness?

The human perception of pain varies over an astounding range. One person may writhe in agony after simply pulling a hamstring while another walks calmly to a phone after having an arm torn off by a piece of farm machinery. Does the injured farmhand produce more endorphins than the hamstring puller, or does he possess a different psychological makeup? Or do both hormonal and psychological factors play a role? If science could uncover why some people seem impervious to pain, we might be able to train others to better handle their otherwise incurable pain. Then we wouldn't have to worry about relieving their pain; we could just teach them to coexist with it. To understand the origins of stoicism, we must decipher that delicate symbiosis between the human mind and physical pain. The answer to "unscientific" pain cures, like herbs and magnets, may likewise reside in that symbiosis.

I have previously mentioned the association of pain and psychiatric disease. Even discounting all the insurance malingerers in the world, we must admit that the mind can manufacture pain de novo in the absence of any bodily infirmity. If that's so, can we achieve the reverse? Can we make the mind create *painlessness* out of thin air, too, despite the presence of painful disease? Lobotomy and cingulotomy come closest to achieving this but demand a steep price. In their place we can try antidepressants, lithium, neuroleptic (antischizophrenic) drugs, antiepileptic drugs, and sedatives, combined with biofeedback, psychotherapy, and behavior modification to achieve a certain degree of psychological pain desensitization. Sometimes it works; often it does not. In general, the best we can hope to accomplish with these psychoactive therapies is the relief of concurrent emotional dysfunctions that may interfere negatively with the perception of true physical pain, like depression, neurosis, or obsessive-compulsive behavior.

A more direct way to alter the perception of pain is to do what Paracelsus advocated centuries ago: appeal to our imaginations. Convince the patient a cure exists, even if it's only an illusion, and he will be cured. I think that's what alternative medicine tries to do. The thing that finally cured Jack, at least in his own mind, was an alternative therapy: a magnetized acupressure back brace.

I must admit here that I dislike the term *alternative therapy* since it implies that there are two types of pain therapy: regular and alternative. In fact, there should only be one class of pain therapies: those that strive to relieve a patient's pain as completely as humanly possible while at the same time keeping the patient's risk, inconvenience, and cost to a minimum. Whether the therapies derive from hard medical science, New Age mysticism, or Haitian voodoo becomes inconsequential. They must work and work safely. This is a point lost on both conventional physicians like me (known as allopathic physicians) and on alternative practitioners. In pain medicine, if it works, it works; if it doesn't, it doesn't. Theory means little to people in pain.

Historically, many so-called alternative methods are as old as allopathic therapies, sometimes even older. In most sciences, old theories tend to be wrong theories—the flat-earth model is older than the round-earth model. In the public's mind, however, old medical therapies tend to be viewed less skeptically than "newfangled" ones. The methods incorporated into Jack's brace, acupuncture and magnetic therapy, are among the oldest forms of medical therapy of any kind. Acupuncture began over two thousand years ago, and magnetic therapy traces back to the fifteenth century and our old friend Paracelsus.

Paracelsus, an avowed alchemist as well as physician, believed that magnets could pull pain out of the body like so much unwanted iron. Fanciful theories notwithstanding, Paracelsus acknowledged that his methods may have succeeded simply because his patients wanted them to succeed. As he relates in the quote at the beginning of this chapter, Paracelsus realized that imagination can be a strong weapon against disease.

Interest in magnetic therapy was rekindled in the eighteenth century thanks to the invention of synthetic permanent magnets with much greater potency than the natural lodestones used by Paracelsus. Interestingly, magnets are like the Rosetta stones of alternative medicine, providing a common link among many different types of alternative medical practices. Franz Mesmer (1734–1815), who would later achieve fame as a hypnotist, stunned Europe by claiming to have cured a woman's mental illness with magnets alone. He proposed a theory of "animal magnetism" in which every creature possesses a magnetic fluid that can be manipulated for therapeutic purposes. In nineteenth-century America, the banner of magnetic therapy was taken up by Daniel David Palmer, who in 1890 founded the Palmer School for Magnetic Cure in Iowa. Palmer combined magnetic therapy with a manual manipulation of the spine of his own invention and called his therapy chiropractic from the Greek word for "hand," *chiros*. Chiropractic, hypnotism, and magnetic therapy persist as alternative pain therapies to the present day.

Although very powerful magnetic fields can influence animal tissues, the strength of popular magnetized bracelets, necklaces, and spinal braces is far too inadequate to produce any medical effect. Moreover, the depth of magnetic penetration created by therapeutic magnets—less than a fraction of an inch—proves that they could not have any effect on underlying joints or muscles. To see how shallow a magnetic field can be, try using a refrigerator magnet to hold up two or three sheets of paper at a time. The magnet can penetrate one piece of paper, but rarely more than one. Thus, it seems clear that magnets can have no biological effect.

Nevertheless, a study performed at the Baylor College of Medicine concluded that magnets significantly reduced the pain of post-polio syndrome, a severe denervation pain occuring in polio victims decades after their initial infection. Curiously, even patients who wore no magnets—but thought they did—got better. The power of imagination was clearly at work here.

⇌

Along with magnets and chiropractic, herbal therapies and acupuncture have also increased in popularity. Herbs are so popular that they now represent the most favored alternative medical therapy (at least in terms of dollars spent). I have no serious quarrel with them, since they are largely (although not entirely) harmless. Pain relievers can be found in the many natural sources—aspirin from willow bark, morphine from poppy seeds, acetaminophen from coal tar. The natural world teems with medicinal compounds.

As for acupuncture, the World Health Organization estimates that there are now ten thousand acupuncturists in the United States alone, almost a third of whom also hold M.D. degrees. In 1993 the U.S. Food and Drug Administration (FDA) estimated that a million Americans made between nine and twelve million visits to an acupuncturist, spending almost $500 million in the process.

Acupuncture postulates that the body contains patterns of energy flow, called Qi (pronounced "chee"), which can be redirected by inserting needles into key acupuncture points on the body, thereby optimizing the patient's health and well-being. The growing popularity of acupuncture in the West can be traced to several pivotal events. The acupuncture ball first got rolling after Richard Nixon's visit to China in 1972, when *New York Times* reporter James Reston described how Chinese physicians relieved his postoperative abdominal pain using acupuncture needles. In the 1990s the FDA declared that acupuncture needles were no longer experimental devices. Finally, in 1997 a consensus panel of the National Institutes of Health, operating under the auspices of the newly created Office of Alternative Medicine (OAM), found that acupuncture might be a useful adjunct to allopathic medicine for certain conditions, including chemotherapy nausea, headache, menstrual cramping, fibromyalgia, low back pain, and carpal tunnel syndrome. Some critics thought that the OAM panel contained too many "pro-acupuncture" members, but there seems little doubt that acupuncture does produce some benefit in selected pain patients.

Some skeptics argue that alternative medical approaches, as a group, yield only placebo responses. I'm not sure this is true. Some techniques, like acupuncture and chiropractic, may also exploit the pain-masking pathways first discovered by Melzack and Wall. Herbal therapies may have a pharmacological basis, and stress reduction techniques like Lamaze and biofeedback may activate the endorphin pathways. But even if the results are only placebo in nature, it remains to be seen whether this is entirely bad. As Paracelsus said, sometimes it's only "the idea" that something will cure pain that counts.

But what exactly is the placebo effect? The word *placebo* literally means "I shall please" and is used to describe treatments that should have no effect at all. Placebos are dummy therapies that have been intentionally designed to appear useful to the patient. If I want to test a new drug, I administer it to half of my patients and give the other half a dummy drug, consisting of sugar or some other relatively inert substance that has been configured to look like the real thing. The placebo has to resemble the real drug, otherwise patients might be biased in reporting their outcomes. In virtually every disease ever studied by placebo-controlled trials, a large number of patients (typically 40 to 50 percent) will report clinical improvement after using placebo drugs or therapies. This is the placebo effect.

It's tempting to dismiss the placebo effect as wishful thinking or delusion, but that would be wrong. The placebo effect occurs so uniformly in so many different populations that it must represent some fundamental property of our mind-body interface. We know that the placebo effect runs deeper than simple psychology, since it can affect things normally beyond our conscious control. For example, placebo drugs can lower blood pressure, raise the heart rate, and even alter the immune response, illustrating how our conscious belief in a dummy treatment can influence subconscious physiological processes. The placebo effect is, of course, a product of the imagination, but imagining is a neurological process that is wired, in turn, to other neurological processes.

We don't yet know the precise biological basis of the placebo effect in pain patients—the precise way that imagination interacts with the physical body. One theory contends that placebo pain control stems from the release of brain opioids; one study showed that the relief of dental pain by the injection of simple saline can be blocked by the drug naltrexone, which neutralizes endogenous endorphins. Another theory argues that the placebo effect derives from a reduction in a patient's expectation of pain and a lowering of general anxiety. In other words, placebos produce pain relief in the same way that Lamaze training reduces obstetric pain: by reducing neurological fear responses that can negatively affect pain perception.

We do know that a placebo's effect on pain can be heightened by a number of factors, including the patient's degree of belief in the treatment and the amount of confidence and enthusiasm displayed by those administering the treatment. People skeptical of chiropractic will be less likely to see a placebo benefit from it; a confident, enthusiastic acupuncturist will obtain more placebo cures than one who appears apathetic. Thus, good outcomes observed after alternative medical therapies may reflect the conjunction of a particularly susceptible patient population with health care providers not known for doubting their wares. One of the reasons why allopathic physicians like myself may fail is that we, as scientists, know that some people will not respond to our therapies and we convey this doubt to our patients. An acupuncturist may succeed where I can't simply because he or she seems so utterly certain that a therapy will work that the patient becomes convinced it cannot fail. If our patients can't imagine a good result, they won't experience a good result.

Jack's belief in the power of magnets was strong. He admitted that he almost tripped over his own feet in his haste to order a magnetized back brace. I don't think he ever ran with the same enthusiasm to my office or to his physical therapy appointments. Thus, Jack was a prime candidate for the placebo effect. The brace was treating his imagination, not his spine. But then, treating his imagination may be therapy enough.

&

A common thread running through many common alternative medical therapies is some form of life force that courses through our bodies and that must be restored or redirected in order to achieve maximum health. In chiropractic it's called spinal energy; in magnetic theory, animal magnetism; in acupuncture, Qi. This concept carries over into certain New Age therapies, where "love" becomes the life-giving force. Although such mysticism would seem a poor analgesic, recall that Joan of Arc smiled as she burned to death. These therapies may tap into a very ancient part of our imagination, a part dealing with mystic beliefs that may be as ancient as the perception of pain itself.

The theories behind chiropractic, acupuncture, therapeutic touch, Native American chanting, and other quasi-mystical pain therapies have been dismissed by the mainstream as mumbo jumbo, when, in fact, they may work precisely because they have a certain supernatural flavor. Most alternative pain therapies require some degree of "magical thinking" in order to inflame the imagination. If I establish a clinic to take peanut butter out of a commercial jar and spread it onto arthritic joints for no good reason, I will get nowhere. On the other hand, if I keep the peanut butter in an exotic apothecary jar and tell patients that it's a plant extract prepared according to a recipe found on an ancient Egyptian papyrus, I will see at least a pronounced placebo effect. The link between magical thinking and pain relief is a well-known but poorly studied phenomenon, a phenomenon that I believe has some basis in neurophysiology.

Finally, C. S. Lewis, in *The Problem of Pain*, notes: "The possibility of pain is inherent in the very existence of a world where souls meet. When souls become wicked they will certainly use this possibility to hurt one another; and this, perhaps, accounts for four-fifths of the sufferings of men. It is men, not God, who have produced racks, whips, prisons, slavery, guns, bayonets, and bombs; it is by human avarice or human stupidity, not by the churlishness of nature, that we have poverty and overwork." Lewis argues that the lion's share of humanity's global pain burden has been placed there by us, not by disease. Just as the source of suffering lies in humanity, the cure for suffering may be found in our humanity as well. The human dimension of pain therapy may also explain some of the public's thirst for unconventional therapies.

Opiates, stimulators, and other scientific therapies are all well and good, but the best therapies are those rendered with liberal doses of attentiveness and kindness, regardless of their underlying mechanism of action. Healers of all stripes must remember that suffering is subjective and, as such, can be modified by subjective things. True, there may be little science behind acupuncture, but an acupuncture treatment requires the practitioner to spend hours attending to the patient, touching the patient, talking to the patient. Chiropractic requires a similar prolonged physical bonding between healer and patient. Through this intimate experience, the acupuncturist enters the imagination and creates a powerful illusion of caring. Although phoning in a prescription for narcotics has greater scientific validity than a trip to the massage therapist, it conjures up none of the healing imagery and physical contact critical for the recovery of chronic pain patients.

So we must still pay heed to the ancient lesson of Paracelsus: Treat the body, but don't underestimate the power of the imagination.

EPILOGUE
Climbing the Mountain

I must die. But must I die groaning? I must be imprisoned.
But must I whine as well? I must suffer exile. Can any one
then hinder me from going with a smile, and a good
courage, and at peace? "Tell the secret." I refuse to
tell.... "But I will chain you." What say you, fellow?
Chain me? My bit of a body, you mean....

—Epictetus (A.D. 55–135)

In 490 B.C. Persia mounted an assault on Greece. When the Greeks finally repelled the Persian invaders, their jubilant commander, Militiades, immediately dispatched a messenger to report his glad tidings to the people of Athens. According to legend, Militiades chose a swift runner named Pheidippides. Pheidippides ran the twenty-six miles between Militiades' headquarters in Marathon and Athens at breakneck speed, and after breathlessly telling the news of victory, promptly dropped dead of exertion. In honor of Pheidippides, modern Olympians run twenty-six-mile "marathons" imitating his feat.

The idea of a healthy person running to the point of death sounds like historical hyperbole, but let's fast-forward time to the present century. The place? The Summer Olympics at Los Angeles in 1984. I remember the spectacle of an exhausted female marathon runner entering the Olympic stadium for her final four hundred meters. Delirious from dehydration and staggering about on cramping legs barely able to support her weight, she careened wildly about the track as though she might collapse and expire at any moment. Officials and spectators alike watched with a mixture of horror and awe as she summoned what little reserves of will and strength she had left and trudged inexorably to a finish line that must have seemed light-years away.

I don't even recall her name—she didn't win any medals or set any records. Victory over other runners wasn't her goal at the end. The crowd that day saw a competition between a woman and her own failing body, a war between human determination and human pain. Amazingly, no one helped her until she crossed the finish line. Maybe they sensed that this form of competition has an inviolate sacredness of its own. She finished the race and was taken to a waiting hospital, where she quickly recovered.

Here, at the end of our own marathon run through the world of pain, I relate the stories of Pheidippides and his modern successor to illustrate what may be the most important lesson of all: We needn't be slaves to pain. Consider the agonies endured by the female marathoner at the end of her race; remember that she *chose* to put herself through that agony. No one threatened her. She didn't run to save her life, or to rescue her children, or to gather food. She ran far beyond where her endorphins could shield her from the pain. She ran to the point of cannibalizing her own muscles and starving her own brain. I have no doubt that if the finish line had been another fifty meters away, she would have willingly perished in the effort, as Pheidippides had done many centuries earlier. In the pursuit of abstract goals—finishing an Olympic marathon and notifying fellow citizens of a great victory—these runners endured supreme torment to the point of collapse and death. And they both succeeded in their goals. There has never been another animal species alive who would suffer so greatly for an ideal.

Although other animals will not turn away from pain if it means survival for themselves or their young, humans often suffer for no reason other than to prove that suffering cannot defeat them. I saw a pro hockey player have four teeth knocked out early in a game and play for another two hours, sucking cold rink air over his bleeding tooth sockets without quitting. Dallas running back Emmitt Smith dislocated a shoulder during a game and never told anyone for fear that he would be made to sit on the bench. Throughout history, soldiers have dashed onto the same battlefields where, only moments earlier, comrades had been dismembered or disemboweled before their eyes. In all of these instances, the body screams, "This hurts, stay away," and the mind ignores the warning. This behavior is neither insane nor masochistic; it is common human behavior that we are all capable of. What pain we choose to ignore depends upon what mountains we want to climb and how badly we want to reach the top.

Recently I had the honor of attending a reception for Sir Edmund Hillary, the New Zealand mountaineer who made history in the 1950s when he became the first person to reach the summit of Mount Everest. Sir Edmund recounted the night before the final assault on the peak, when he and his Sherpa guide, Tensing Norgay, dug beds in the thick snow and pitched a flimsy tent at the foot of the last remaining ice wall. They were so short of breath that they couldn't sleep unless they consumed some of their precious oxygen supply; they finally settled on sleeping for only three hours in order to conserve oxygen for the rigorous climb ahead. With temperatures well below freezing and Everest's notorious winds whipping through their makeshift shelter, Hillary and Norgay huddled in the thin air and wheezed away the hours until dawn. Hillary said that he was more miserable that night than at any time in his life, before or since, but he never gave a thought to turning back. The summit awaited him and that meant more than any pain. Hillary knew that when human *will* confronts human *pain*, will usually triumphs.

Like Hillary, we all have personal mountains to scale. By keeping our eyes fixed on the summit, we can look past pain. And our mountains don't have to be Everests. I like to play tennis and practice the martial arts despite the pains of an aging body— small mountains to be sure, but they enable me to endure. Whether entering combat, running for glory, or testing for a black belt in a local shopping mall, we can accept and ignore pain in the pursuit of a goal. We can deal better with pain that has a purpose, a significance, a meaning.

This explains why so many chronic pain patients descend into deep despair: their pain is devoid of meaning. They have a suffering that's without purpose, a pain both sterile and pointless. They have the pain of hell—utterly useless—while Hillary's pain was of purgatory, a physical price to be paid for a meta-physical reward. The boxer takes years of facial beatings in ex-change for a championship belt, but the trigeminal neuralgia patient gets beaten sans cheering fans. A career weight lifter en-dures aching joints as the price of a gorgeous body, but the rheumatoid arthritis patient doesn't trade pain for bulging muscles. The boxer and weight lifter may even endure more pain in their lifetimes than people with actual diseases, but their pain has tangible value.

People often look for religion to give meaning to otherwise meaningless torment. If sufferers can't achieve an earthly goal with their torment, a supernatural goal, like heaven or reincarna-tion into a better life, will do. When the late Mother Teresa first began ministering to the untouchable Hindus in Calcutta, she en-countered resistance—from the Hindus themselves. Their incredible suffering had value to them; it permitted them to escape their untouchable status in the next cycle of life. If they enjoyed themselves too much in the present life, they would have to be born again into another miserable existence later. For them, starvation and disease served the same role as a tough fraternity hazing, a punishment they took gladly so as to achieve membership in a higher caste after death.

The biblical blueprint for understanding pointless pain is found in the Book of Job. Job, a wealthy (but pious) man, lost his family, fortune, and health for no reason save the caprice of the Almighty. God rewarded Job later for Job's refusal to blame God during his torment. The lesson of Job? That all pain has a purpose. We may not know or understand what that purpose is, but we shouldn't question that it exists. To the religious, God has given us the mountains to climb. For some, the climb is easy; for others, quite difficult. But a worthy summit exists for all who suffer, whether they see it plainly or not. In Job's case, suffering was merely a test of loyalty.

❧

The opening quote from the Stoic philosopher Epictetus reflects the importance of attitude in dealing with pain. At first reading, it sounds like something from a glib pop philosopher—if we're going to suffer, at least suffer with a smile. But Epictetus goes on to make a more profound point later: You can chain me, he says, but you can only chain my "bit" of a body. In other words, pain affects only our physical bodies and our bodies are but a small dimension of our being. Pain can chain our bodies but can never chain our minds unless we permit it to do so. If we study all the triumphs of the human psyche over great diseases and injury, we will see that the body is indeed the lesser partner in the mind-body dualism. Epictetus knew the lesson of lobotomy two thousand years before we did: how we perceive pain psychologically, our attitude toward pain, makes all the difference in the world.

When medicines and operations, magnets and chiropractors all fail (and that happens far too frequently), chronic pain patients may yet save themselves from falling into a void, by looking for some point to their pain, some *meaning*. They have to envision pain not as the end, but as the means; not as hell, but as purgatory. For Edmund Hillary, suffering was a means to the top of the world; for the marathon runner, a means to the finish line. But how can this state of mind be achieved? No blanket formula can be devised, but I've seen many people succeed on a case-by-case basis.

For some, the search for meaning draws them closer to their gods and their religions. For others, a more earthbound approach works well: volunteering to help other people with the same affliction; participating in medical trials; raising money or lecturing to cure a disease or promote public understanding. I knew one woman with intractable face pain who enjoyed counseling other victims of face pain so much that she began to see her own illness in a different light. Without personally experiencing the disease, she would never have had the opportunity to minister to others. She found meaning in an otherwise meaningless malady and came to see it as a blessing. In a sense, she was cured, not by craniotomy but by a restructuring of her attitude.

Why do we hurt? Because despite all of our ethereal properties, humankind has not yet slipped the bonds of our mortal bodies. Gibbon once said of ancient Rome that it was destined to die from the "injuries of time," and so are we. Death becomes our ultimate analgesic, but we shouldn't embrace it lightly. As Epictetus said so long ago, we don't have to let the body's chains weigh down our spirits, too. We must try to shed the chains of pain, cloak our souls against the cold, and continue to climb our mountains.

So I have one last bit of advice for those in pain: Envision your personal finish line and keep going forward. And don't rely completely on those around you to be your salvation. Like the marathon runner, you may have to stagger home alone. After all, the struggle to wrest our lives free of pain's bondage must be fought, first and last, within ourselves.

INDEX